Clinical Skills Manual for Pediatric Nursing

Caring for Children

THIRD EDITION

Ruth C. Bindler, RNC, PhD

Associate Professor, Intercollegiate College of Nursing
Washington State University
Spokane, Washington

Jane W. Ball, RN, CPNP, DrPH

Executive Director, Emergency Medical Services for Children
National Resource Center, Children's National Medical Center
Washington, D.C.

Prentice Hall

Upper Saddle River, NJ 07458

Publisher: Julie Levin Alexander
Assistant to Publisher: Regina Bruno
Executive Editor: Maura Connor
Senior Managing Editor: Marilyn Meserve
Development Editor: Kim Wyatt
Assistant Editor: Yesenia Kopperman
Editorial Assistant: Sladjana Repic
Director of Production and Manufacturing: Bruce Johnson
Managing Production Editor: Patrick Walsh
Production Liaison: Danielle Newhouse
Production Editor: Lori Dalberg, Carlisle Publishers Services
Manufacturing Manager: Ilene Sanford
Design Director: Cheryl Asherman
Design Coordinator: Maria Guglielmo
Interior Designer: Wanda España
Cover Designer: Cheryl Asherman
Electronic Art Creation: Precision Graphics
Photographers: Roy Ramsey
Marketing Manager: Nicole Benson
Marketing Coordinator: Janet Ryerson
Production Information Manager: Rachele Strober
Composition: Carlisle Communications, Ltd.
Cover Printer: Phoenix Color
Printing and Binding: Banta Menasha

Pearson Education, Ltd.
Pearson Education Australia Pty., Limited
Pearson Education Singapore, Pte. Ltd.
Pearson Education North Asia Ltd.
Pearson Education Canada Ltd.
Pearson Educación de Mexico, S.A. de C.V.
Pearson Education — Japan
Pearson Education Malaysia, Pte. Ltd.

10 9 8 7 6 5 4 3 2
ISBN 0-13-048352-4

Contents

CHAPTER 6

Specimen Collection   39

CHAPTER 7

Administration of Medication 51

CHAPTER 11

Nutrition   115

CHAPTER 12

Elimination   123

CHAPTER 13

Musculoskeletal Care   129

Preface

Writing a skills manual is a constantly evolving process. Technology and techniques change and new research leads to new procedures. Thus, we are constantly revising and improving the information presented here, material that we now find is in demand. Although the *Clinical Skills Manual* is designed to be an independent skills procedure manual, it began as an accompaniment to the textbook *Pediatric Nursing: Caring for Children.* For the first edition of the text, skills information was placed as an appendix within the text. In the second edition, a separate quick reference to pediatric skills was packaged with the text so that students could more easily carry the reference to clinical settings. Because practicing nurses and others sought extra copies of the manual for use in clinical settings, the skills manual has been expanded and revised so that it can stand on its own as an independent reference for students and nurses alike.

Organization and Overview

Performance of clinical skills is one of the essential components of successful nursing care. Skills can be challenging to perform on children due to their differing levels of growth and development, lack of ability to communicate or understand information about procedures, and some differences from techniques in adults. The clinical skills manual was designed to assist practitioners in the safe performance of skills commonly performed on children.

The skills are presented concisely to emphasize essential information. It is assumed that students have had a basic course in skill procedures, so this reference is designed to emphasize pediatric variations. Skills are grouped into chapters that reflect a type of intervention. Chapters begin with those that are foundational to nursing care, branching out into those that are grouped by system or skill set. Each skill begins with a short description, followed by the **preparation** needed by the nurse, **equipment and supplies** required, and the **procedure**. **Rationale** is inserted within the presentations to explain the reason for certain preparations and procedures.

Several approaches are used to assist the student in understanding and carrying out the skills. Photographs provide a visual image of equipment and technique. Margin boxes and tables highlight important safety issues, growth and development considerations, teaching for families, and clinical tips. Students using the textbook *Pediatric Nursing* will find icons inserted that indicate when a skill has been described in the skills manual. The student can thus move between these two resources to apply theoretical knowledge readily in the clinical setting.

The clinical skills manual ends with appendices that provide information on growth grids and calculation of body surface area for medication administration. The book is compact so that it can easily be used by students and nurses in the clinical area.

NOTE: Students and nurses should consult their hospital or institution procedure manual or other references for more detailed and specific information when needed.

Changes to the Third Edition

Due to interest from nurses in a variety of pediatric disciplines, all of the skills content has been updated and expanded from the previous version. Over two dozen new skills have been added, rationales have been indicated throughout all procedures, and 25 new color photographs help illustrate techniques and equipment.

Acknowledgments

This clinical skills manual has become a reality through the dedication and hard work of many individuals. First we would like to acknowledge the vision of Maura Connor, our editor at Prentice Hall Health, who supported the idea of a separate and expanded skills manual. Photographs for the former and present editions were taken by George Dodson and Roy Ramsey. Both of these talented individuals are sensitive to issues related to children and families in clinical settings and are creative and proficient in capturing the images of children and nurses. Connie Boleneus provided support and expertise in the photography in a practice laboratory. Our developmental editor, Kim Wyatt, helped us greatly with organization of content, cohesive flow of material, and in making the vision for the manual a reality. Editorial Assistant Sladjana Repic was essential in facilitating communications with Prentice Hall; her pleasant and competent manner were outstanding. We thank Danielle Newhouse, production editor, Patrick Walsh, production managing editor, and Nicole Benson, senior marketing manager, for their valuable contributions. Our thanks also go to Cheryl Asherman, design director, for creating the design. At Carlisle Communications, we thank Lori Dalberg for coordinating production. We acknowledge as well the contributions of individuals to past editions of the manual. Marcia Wellington, Jane Novoa, Karen Frank, and Neysa Dobson assisted by providing material and feedback for prior editions.

Ruth C. Bindler
Jane W. Ball

Reviewers

Phoenix Children's Hospital

Louise Aurilio, PhD, MSN, RNC, CNA
Youngstown State University
Girard, OH

Kathaleen C. Bloom, PhD, CNM
University of North Florida
Jacksonville, FL

Constance Bobik, RN, BSN, MSN
Brevard Community College
Titusville, FL

Judy Buzby RN
Niagara County Community College
Sanborn, NY

Cheryl DeGraw RN, MSN, CRNP
Florence Darlington Technical College
Florence, SC

Lisa Haynie, RN, MSN, CFNP
University of Mississippi School of Nursing
Jackson, MS

LaDonna K. Northington RN, DNS
University of Mississippi School of Nursing
Jackson, MS

Roselle Partridge, RNC, MSN
Indiana University School of Nursing
Indianapolis, IN

Sharon A. Vinten RNC, MSN, WHNP
Indiana University School of Nursing
Indianapolis, IN

P. Renee Williams, RN, MSN, CCE
University of Mississippi School of Nursing
Jackson, MS

Student Reviewers

Michele Berkstresser
University of Scranton
Bridgewater, NJ

Debra Brooks
University of Scranton
Scranton, PA

Introduction

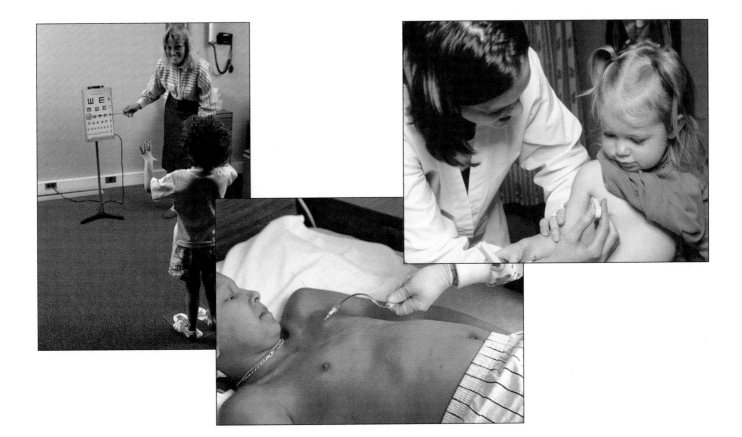

Nurses often perform procedures on children in homes, clinics, and hospitals. These procedures, although similar to those performed on adults, differ in several ways. Nurses must therefore be knowledgeable about skills common in child health settings, as well as understanding variations in preparation, equipment, and techniques needed to perform skills on children. The nurse also integrates knowledge of health promotion and disease prevention by performing screening in children.

General Guidelines

Preparation for procedures must taken into account a child's developmental stage and cognitive ability. *General guidelines for preparing the child* and are outlined below.

- Review the technique as needed.
- Explain the procedure to the child and family in a manner they can understand.
- Verify understanding and ask if they have questions about the procedure.
- Inquire if the parent wishes to be present and if the child (when old enough) wants the parent present.
- Obtain consent for the procedure if needed.
- Obtain necessary equipment and supplies.

Children are taken to a treatment room or to another room for potentially painful or frightening procedures. The child's room and the playroom are thus kept as "safe" areas in which painful procedures are not performed. If parents wish to be present they can be helped to support the child. When possible, it is best to have other personnel restrain the child or assist with the procedure so that the child does not view the parent as causing the discomfort.

When a skill is to be performed on a child, *general guidelines for performing the procedure* include:

- Check the medical order to verify the procedure.
- Identify the child by name band and/or other identification.
- Verify that the consent is signed if needed.
- Greet the parent and child.
- Give explanations and instructions about the specific plan to the child and parent.
- Wash your hands.
- Prepare necessary equipment.

- Don gloves as needed.
- Perform the procedure.
- Clean the area as needed.
- Document the performance of the procedure and results.

There are two major concerns the nurse should keep in mind when performing procedures on children. These include *safety* and *comfort*. The nurse ensures that correct procedures are followed so that the child is kept free from harm. Approaches should be used to promote understanding and comfort for both the child and parents. Nurses play a vital role in skill performance that enhances diagnosis and treatment of children in many settings.

1

Informed Consent

Chapter Outline

General Guidelines for Obtaining Informed Consent

Informed consent involves explaining a specific procedure to the parent (or legal guardian) or to the patient and then obtaining written permission to perform the specific procedure.

Before a procedure, the parent or legal guardian and patient (to the level of the child's ability) must be given enough information to clearly understand the condition, a detailed description of the procedure or treatment to be performed, the possible benefits and significant risks associated with the procedure or treatment involved, and alternative methods available to achieve the same end. The parent or guardian is also informed of the right to refuse treatment on behalf of the child.

It is both legally and ethically necessary to obtain informed consent. Without signed permission for medical management, the physician, nurse, or other health care provider could be found guilty of assault and battery.

Guidelines have been established to ensure that informed consent is obtained for medical care. Additional guidelines are available when performing research on children, and this information can be found in Chapter 1 of *Pediatric Nursing, Caring for Children, Third Edition.*

- Information must be presented to individuals who are responsible for making an informed decision to allow them the opportunity to weigh the benefits of the proposed treatment or procedure against the potential for complications. This information should be presented in simple, easy-to-understand terms. All questions and concerns should be answered honestly. If necessary, an interpreter should be used to ensure clear communication.
- The decision maker must be over the age of majority (i.e., the age at which full civil rights are accorded—18 years in most states) and must be competent (i.e., must be able to make a decision based on the information received). The person needs to understand the proposed medical management and any risks. In some states, adolescents between the ages of 13 and 18 are able to sign for some treatment alone (e.g., birth control, substance abuse treatment). Know the parameters of the state law where you practice nursing.
- The decision reached must be voluntary. The person making the decision must not be coerced, forced, under medication that can influence judgment, or placed under duress while considering the options.

Although general written consent for care is obtained within the hospital setting during the admission process, specific consent must be obtained for the following procedures or treatments:

- Major surgery
- Minor surgery such as a cutdown, incision and drainage, closed reduction of a fracture, or fracture pinning
- Invasive diagnostic tests such as lumbar puncture, bone marrow aspiration, biopsy, cardiac catheterization, or endoscopy
- Treatments that may involve high risk, such as radiation therapy, chemotherapy, or dialysis
- Any procedure or treatment that falls under the auspices of research
- Photographing patients, even when done for educational purposes

SKILL 1-1 Pediatric Considerations for Obtaining Informed Consent

PREPARATION

1. Assess the parent's knowledge about the procedure so that during the discussion with the physician correct information can be reinforced and misconceptions can be clarified.

2. Assess the child's ability to understand information and participate in the decision-making process.
   - *If the child is a minor* (has not reached the age of majority—under the age of 18 years in most states), the child's parent or legal guardian must give consent for all procedures or treatments. *Mature minors* (e.g., adolescents aged 14 to 15 who are able to understand treatment risks) can give consent for treatment or refuse treatment in some states. Children should become more actively involved in decision making about treatment procedures as their reasoning skills develop. Children too young to give informed consent can be given age-appropriate information about their condition and asked about their care preferences. Their parents, however, make ultimate decisions regarding their care.

     RATIONALE: *By age 14, an adolescent can weigh options and make decisions regarding consent as capably as an adult. By 7 or 8 years of age, a child is able to understand concrete explanations about informed consent for research participation. By age 11, a child's abstract reasoning and logic are advanced.*

   - Some states provide for the rights of nonemancipated teens to make certain health care decisions. The child may give permission only for those conditions identified in state law, and only at the ages specified by that particular state. Some examples of the treatments for which many states permit an adolescent's signature include birth control, treatment of sexually transmitted infections, contraceptive and abortion counseling and services, substance abuse, and mental illness (Muscari, 1998). Check the law in your state for guidelines.

   - *If the child is an emancipated minor* (under the age of 18 who is legally independent), the child may give informed consent for medical care. Common examples of emancipated minors include teenagers who are married, in the military, living apart from their parents and financially independent, or are pregnant or parents themselves.

3. If a parent or guardian is not available, determine that an authorized adult can give informed consent.
   - When a parent or guardian is unavailable to provide consent for treatment, the person in charge of the child (e.g., relative, baby-sitter, teacher, or camp counselor) may give consent for emergency treatment if the person has signed, written permission from the parent or guardian to authorize care in his or her absence. When the parent or guardian can be contacted by telephone, verbal consent can be obtained with two witnesses listening simultaneously. The consent should be recorded for later signature. Under federal law Emergency Medical Treatment and Labor Act (EMTALA), a minor can be examined, treated, stabilized, and even transferred to another hospital for emergency care without consent ever being obtained from the parent or legal guardian (Bitterman, 2000).

EQUIPMENT AND SUPPLIES

- Private area
- Appropriate forms and educational materials
- Pen

PROCEDURE

1. Notify the physician that the family is available to discuss the procedure.

2. Obtain necessary forms and written explanations of procedure.

3. Find a quiet place where the physician and nurse can explain the forms and procedure to the child and/or family.

4. Accompany the physician to serve as a witness and to assist with answering the family's questions.

   RATIONALE: *The nurse's role is to serve as a witness for the physician that the family was fully informed about the procedure and their right to consent to or refuse treatment. The nurse also assists by ensuring that the information provided by the physician is understood by the family and put into a context that has meaning to the family.*

5. Ask family members several questions to evaluate their understanding. Provide additional information when any points must be clarified.

6. When family members appear to have no more questions, ask if they are prepared to give consent for the procedure or need more time to consider the options.

7. When family members are prepared to give consent, obtain their signatures and serve as a witness to their consent.

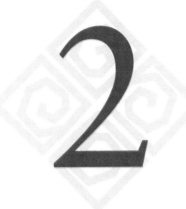

Positioning and Restraint

Chapter Outline

Guidelines for the use of mechanical and chemical restraints for children should exist in all health care facilities. The Joint Commission on Accreditation of Health Care Organizations (JCAHO) has specific standards with regard to the use of restraints. In general, restraints must be prescribed, and guidelines for how frequently the child must be removed from the restraints should be stated.

A preferred method of restraint is to have a trained person be present with a child so that observation can replace mechanical or chemical restraint when possible. For example, when a child must be held in position for a procedure, it is important to try to use an assistant rather than a mechanical restraint for this purpose. Although some parents are comfortable holding their child for a procedure, most prefer to be close and act as a support person and allow health professionals to provide restraint. This allows the parent to be free to provide comfort and to avoid the role of holding the child for a painful or stressful procedure. The child then can view the parent as a solace rather than as someone who brings pain. With the parent nearby, the child will be far less anxious and will not feel that he or she is being punished.

Human Restraint

SKILL 2-1 Positioning a Child for Intravenous Access/Injection

PREPARATION

1. Determine if the parent wants to be present during an uncomfortable procedure or to be available after the procedure to provide comfort.

2. When the parent wishes to be present, discuss the parent's role (e.g., holding the child or providing distraction or comfort during the procedure).

3. Ensure that the person positioning and holding the child (parent or other assistant) clearly understands what body parts must be held still and how to do this safely.

EQUIPMENT AND SUPPLIES

- Supplies for procedure to be performed
- Infection control supplies as needed

PROCEDURE: *Supine Position*

1. Place the child in a supine position on a bed or stretcher.
   RATIONALE: *This position allows the child to see what is happening and thus reduces some of the child's fear.*

2. Have the parent, a nurse, or an assistant lean over the child to restrain the child's body and extend the extremity to be used for access or injection.
   RATIONALE: *The nurse's body provides a source of human contact as well as securing the child so that the procedure can be done quickly.*

Sitting Position

1. Have the child sit on the parent's or assistant's lap with legs held firmly between the assistant's legs. The child's arms can be wrapped around the parent's or assistant's waist.

2. Have the parent or assistant hold the child firmly against the chest, wrapping arms around the child's upper body (Figure 2-1).
   RATIONALE: *This hugging position adds comfort and security so the procedure can be done quickly.*

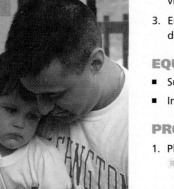

Figure 2-1 *The child should be restrained by the parent or an assistant during intramuscular injection.*

SKILL 2-2 Positioning a Child for Lumbar Puncture

PREPARATION

1. Determine if the parent wants to be present during an uncomfortable procedure or to be available after the procedure to provide comfort.
2. When the parent wishes to be present, discuss the parent's role (e.g., providing distraction or comfort during the procedure).
3. Ensure that the person positioning and holding the child clearly understands what body parts must be held still and how to do this safely.

EQUIPMENT AND SUPPLIES

- Supplies for procedure to be performed
- Infection control supplies as needed

PROCEDURE

1. Place the child on his or her side with knees pulled to the abdomen and the neck flexed to the chin. The assistant can hold the child in position by wrapping one arm behind the knees and the other behind the neck, keeping the back curved.
   RATIONALE: *This position ensures the best possible access to spinal processes and disk spaces.*
2. The *infant* can be held in this position easily by holding the neck and thighs with the hands (Figure 2-2).
3. The *older child* can be quite strong, and someone with enough strength will be needed to hold him or her in this position. Lean over the child with the entire body, using the forearms against the thighs and around the shoulders and head (Figure 2-3).

> **NURSING ALERT**
>
> Lumbar puncture requires that the child be held still to prevent injury and to ensure success at obtaining fluid. It is advisable to have an experienced staff member hold the child in position for the procedure.

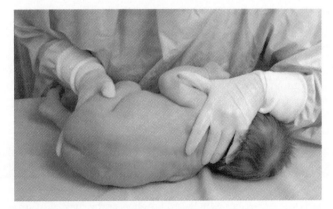

Figure 2-2 *Infant positioned for lumbar puncture.*

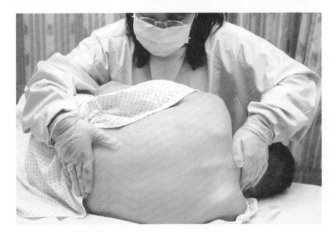

Figure 2-3 *Child positioned for lumbar puncture.*

SKILL 2-3 Positioning a Child for an Otoscopic Examination

PREPARATION

1. Determine if the parent wants to be present during an uncomfortable procedure or to be available after the procedure to provide comfort.
2. When the parent wishes to be present, discuss the parent's role (e.g., holding the child or providing distraction or comfort during the procedure).

3. Ensure that the person positioning and holding the child (parent or other assistant) clearly understands what body parts must be held still and how to do this safely.

EQUIPMENT AND SUPPLIES
- Supplies for procedure to be performed
- Infection control supplies as needed

PROCEDURE: *Supine Position*

1. Place the child in a supine position on a bed or stretcher. Have the parent, a nurse, or an assistant lean over the child to restrain the child's arms and body. The assistant may also assist with stabilizing the child's head.

2. Hold the otoscope in the hand closest to the child's face and, when the child is cooperative, rest the back of the hand against the child's head.
   RATIONALE: *This action provides additional stabilization of the child's head to prevent pain and injury when the otoscope earpiece is inserted into the auditory canal.*

3. Use the other hand to pull the pinna toward the back of the head and either up or down (Figure 2-4).
   RATIONALE: *This action straightens the ear canal so that the tympanic membrane can be visualized.*

Sitting Position

1. Have the child sit on the parent's or assistant's lap with legs held firmly between the assistant's legs. The child's arms can be wrapped around the parent's or assistant's waist.

2. Have the parent or assistant hold the child's head firmly against the chest with one arm while the other arm holds the arms and upper chest.
   RATIONALE: *This position provides comfort to the child while securing the head.*

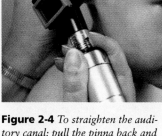

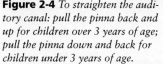

Figure 2-4 *To straighten the auditory canal: pull the pinna back and up for children over 3 years of age; pull the pinna down and back for children under 3 years of age.*

Mechanical Restraint

Temporary mechanical restraints are used to decrease the child's movement and to allow the health care provider to carry out a procedure. It is effective when procedures are being performed on the head, or on an extremity as one limb can be left out for the procedure.

SKILL 2-4 Applying a Papoose Restraint

The papoose consists of a board and cloth wrappings with Velcro fasteners at the chest, hips, and knees (Figure 2-5). Two sizes are available—one for infants and toddlers and one for larger children. Some papooses come with openings for arms. For example, if the child is positioned for a venipuncture, the arm can fit through the opening in the vest and then the remaining fabric pieces can be secured.

PREPARATION

1. Explain the reason for the restraint to the child and parent and how long it will be needed. Tell the child how the restraint will feel.
   RATIONALE: *Young children will be less anxious if the explanation about what they will feel is placed in nonthreatening terms.*

2. Gather equipment and supplies for procedure.
   RATIONALE: *Having supplies prepared reduces the time the child spends in temporary restraint devices and thus the level of anxiety.*

3. Have an assistant (or a parent) available to help restrain a body part if needed.
   RATIONALE: *The papoose is most often used when the nurse has no assistant available or a parent is unwilling to restrain the child for a procedure.*

EQUIPMENT AND SUPPLIES

- Restraint board (papoose) to fit child's size
- Sheet
- Infection control supplies as needed

PROCEDURE

1. Place a towel or sheet over the board.

2. Have the child lie supine on the board, with the head at the top.

3. Place the fabric wrappings around the child, and secure the Velcro fasteners. To be most effective, the fabric wrappings should be secure over the elbows, hips, and knees.

   RATIONALE: *This action prevents the child from pulling apart the wrappings or from kicking.*

4. After the procedure, release the child and allow the parents to provide comfort.

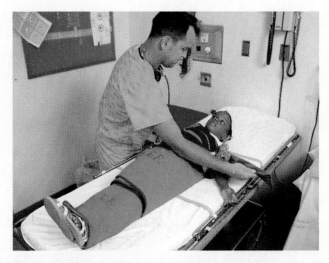

Figure 2-5 *Child on a papoose restraint board.*

SKILL 2-5 Applying a Mummy Restraint

Mummy restraint consists of wrapping the child securely in a blanket or sheet.

PREPARATION

1. Explain the procedure to the child and parent.

2. Have all supplies and materials for the procedure collected and ready for use.

EQUIPMENT AND SUPPLIES

- Soft blanket or sheet 2 to 3 times larger than the child

PROCEDURE: *Infant*

1. Put the blanket (or sheet) on the bed or examination table. Fold down one corner until it reaches the middle of the blanket.

2. Place the infant in a diagonal position with his or her neck on the folded edge.

3. Bring one side of the blanket over the infant's arm and then under the back. Tuck that edge under and over the other arm and around the back.

4. Bring the other side of the blanket around the body and tuck underneath the body.

5. Bring the bottom corner of the blanket up and over the abdomen.

Toddler and Older Child

1. Put the blanket (or sheet) on the bed or examination table. Fold down one corner until it reaches the middle of the blanket.

2. Place the child on the blanket, positioning so that there is sufficient material to wrap the knees and lower legs. If necessary, fold down the top edges of the blanket to the shoulders.

3. Bring one side of the blanket over the arm, body, and legs and tuck it under the other arm and around the back and legs (Figure 2-6A).

4. Bring the other side of the blanket up and around the body, and tuck underneath the back and legs (Figure 2-6B) (Figure 2-6C).

   RATIONALE: *The child should not be able to flex the knees and kick or it may be impossible to perform the procedure.*

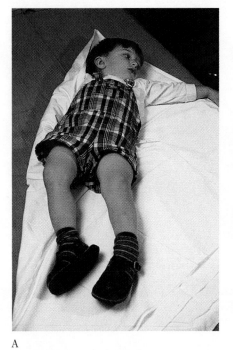

A

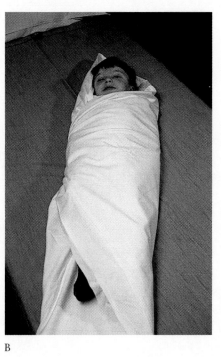

B

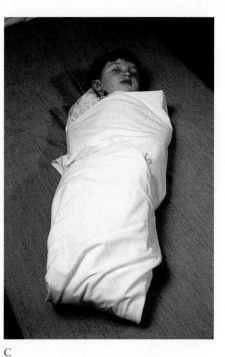

C

Figure 2-6 *Steps in applying a mummy restraint.*

SKILL 2-6 Applying Elbow Restraints

In 1997, the American Academy of Pediatrics established guidelines on the use of physical restraint for children and adolescents in the acute care setting. They recommend:

- Explaining the procedure to the child

- Obtaining a written or verbal order for restraint from the physician, stating the type of restraint and its expected duration

- Providing an immediate explanation to the family about the need for restraint and documenting this in the medical record

- Performing assessment: Is the restraint applied correctly? Are skin and neurovascular status intact? Is the restraint accomplishing its purpose? Is there a need to continue using the restraint?

Elbow restraints (Figure 2-7) are used to prevent the infant or child from reaching his or her face or head, especially after surgery. Because the restraints must be on the child for an extended time, a medical order is required.

PREPARATION

1. Explain the need for the elbow restraints to the parent.

2. Verify the medical order for the restraints. Review the institution's policy for use of restraints and plan the times when the child is released from restraints.

EQUIPMENT AND SUPPLIES

- Ready-made elbow restraints are available commercially.

- An elbow restraint can be devised easily from a piece of muslin that has vertical pockets sewn into it. Tongue depressors are inserted into the pockets.

- Pins or tape

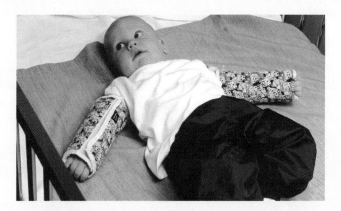

Figure 2-7 *Infant with elbow restraints.*

PROCEDURE

1. Wrap the elbow restraint around the arm from axilla to wrist snug enough to prevent bending of the elbow.

2. Secure the restraint with pins or tape.

3. Remove the elbow restraints at least every 2 hours (or the interval specified in the institution's guidelines).

   RATIONALE: *The restraint may cause skin abrasion or impair circulation if placed too snugly around the arm.*

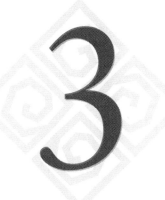

3

Transport

Chapter Outline

Children must often be transported within the health care facility to have tests performed or receive treatments, or be transferred to home or another facility. Safety is the most important aspect of transporting infants and children. In determining the best method of transporting a child, the developmental stage must be taken into consideration. For short transports within the unit, an infant or young child may be carried in an adult's arms; however, for transports off the unit and when the child is older than toddlerhood, transport with cribs or other such equipment is used. For safety, the child should be visible to the transporting adult at all times. The child's comfort must be considered, with measures taken to promote support and comfort. When parents are present they may travel with the child to provide comfort.

> **HOME CARE CONSIDERATIONS**
>
> When the child with medical equipment or casts is going to be discharged, assist the family to plan for car seats and alteration of the home to facilitate the child's needs. See Chapter 21 of *Pediatric Nursing: Caring for Children, Third Edition,* and the accompanying CD for resources to offer parents.

SKILL 3-1 Transport of the Infant

PREPARATION

1. Obtain necessary transporting equipment.

2. Securely fasten intravenous lines, feeding lines, EKG leads, and other equipment.
   RATIONALE: *Lines that are securely fastened are less likely to be dislodged during transport.*

3. Explain the transport plan to the family.
   RATIONALE: *Adequate explanation helps to decrease anxiety.*

EQUIPMENT AND SUPPLIES

- Transporting vehicle (e.g., stretcher, crib, wheel chair)
- Wheeled poles for any necessary equipment
- Blankets

PROCEDURE

1. Perform an assessment of the child.
   RATIONALE: *A baseline assessment provides comparison with later findings. At times, transport may adversely affect the child's condition and initial assessment data provide necessary information.*

2. The infant is placed in a bassinet or crib for transport. If the bassinet has a bottom shelf, it is used for carrying equipment such as an intravenous pump or monitor.

3. Attach intravenous poles and other equipment to the crib. When this is not possible, adequate personnel are needed to push all of the equipment.
   RATIONALE: *Lines can be more easily kept intact if they are on one transport vehicle.*

4. Keep the infant covered with blankets.
   RATIONALE: *Adequate covers help to prevent hypothermia resulting from a cool environment.*

5. Allow parents to accompany the child on the transport when possible.
   RATIONALE: *The parents' presence can provide a sense of security for the young child.*

SKILL 3-2 Transport of the Toddler

PREPARATION

1. Obtain necessary transporting equipment.

2. Securely fasten intravenous lines, feeding lines, EKG leads, and other equipment.

3. Explain the transport plan to the family.

EQUIPMENT AND SUPPLIES

- Transporting vehicle (e.g., stretcher, crib, wheel chair)
- Wheeled poles for any necessary equipment
- Blankets

PROCEDURE

1. Transport the toddler in a high-top crib (also used for infants, and shown in Figure 3-1), with the siderails up and the protective top in place. The child may be sitting or lying down. Alternatively, secure the child in a stroller or wheelchair of the proper size for the child's age.
   RATIONALE: *Stretchers should not be used because the mobile toddler may roll or fall off.*

2. Be sure to secure the child in the device with the seat safety strap (Figure 3-2).
   RATIONALE: *The child is secured to avoid falls and injury during transport.*

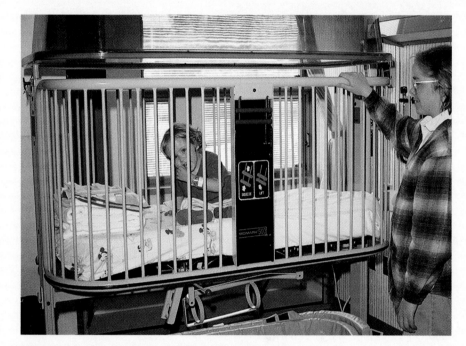

Figure 3-1 *High-top crib for infant of toddler transport.*

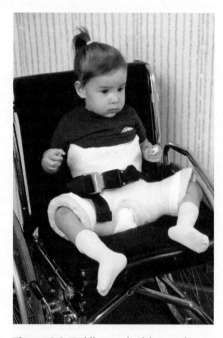

Figure 3-2 *Toddler in wheelchair with safety strap.*

SKILL 3-3   Transport of the Child with Disability

PREPARATION

1. Obtain necessary transporting equipment.
2. Securely fasten intravenous lines, feeding lines, EKG leads, and other equipment.
3. Explain the transport plan to the family.

EQUIPMENT AND SUPPLIES

- Transporting vehicle (e.g., stretcher, crib, wheel chair)
- Wheeled poles for any necessary equipment
- Blankets

PROCEDURE

1. Use a wheelchair or stretcher for the older child who is unable to walk because of a disability or whose mobility must be restricted (Figure 3-3).

2. Secure safety belts and supervise the child closely.

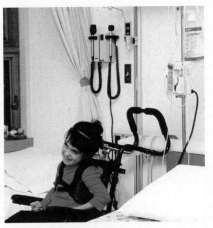

Figure 3-3 *The child who is getting tube feedings or other infusions during the day can easily and safely be transported in a wheelchair with the tube feeding or infusion on a pole. Pumps can also be attached to the pole when used to regulate infusion rates.*

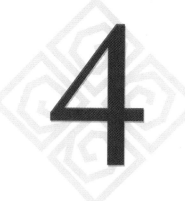

Infection Control Methods

Chapter Outline

Infection Control Methods

CLINICAL TIP

Always use nonlatex gloves if the child has an allergy or sensitivity to latex, or if the health care provider has latex sensitivity. See Chapter 11 of *Pediatric Nursing: Caring for Children, Third Edition,* for information on latex allergy.

Special methods are used to provide infection control. The two levels of precautions are standard control and transmission-based control. Consult the Centers for Disease Control and Prevention (CDC) for details on infection control. Prior to patient contact, decide what type of precautions are needed. Examples are as follows:

- *Masks* protect from pathogens that are shed through respiratory droplets.
- *Gloves* protect the skin from contact with pathogens. Gloves are worn when contact with mucous membranes, nonintact skin, or moist body substances is possible.
  RATIONALE: *Gloves protect both the child and the health care provider from contamination and transferal of infective agents.*

- *Gowns* protect against contact with pathogens when it is likely that body substances will come in contact with the health care provider's clothing. Change gowns between contacts with other patients.
- *Protective eyewear* such as goggles or face shields protect against the risk of blood or body fluid being splattered. Wear them when the eyes, nose, or mouth may be splashed by the patient's body substances and when in close proximity to any open skin lesions.

Standard Precautions

Standard precautions are used in the care of all patients, regardless of diagnoses, when contact with blood, body fluids, secretions, excretions, nonintact skin, mucous membranes, or materials contaminated with these substances might occur. Always have access to protective equipment and add items as needed. The following general guidelines should be used.

1. Wash hands before and after patient contact and when needed during contact.
2. Wear gloves when contact with blood, body fluids, secretions, excretions, nonintact skin, or mucous membranes might occur. Change gloves each time they are contaminated with these substances, washing hands before regloving.
3. Wear additional protective equipment such as gown, mask, and goggles if body fluid splashes can occur.
4. Wear the protective equipment to clean up body fluid spills. Discard waste in appropriate body substance waste containers. Clean the area with bleach or another acceptable cleaner. Bag contaminated laundry in secured and labeled bags.
5. Discard needles, scalpels, and lancets in labeled sharps containers without recapping.
6. Place patients who could contaminate the environment with airborne or droplet infection in private rooms.

Transmission-Based Precautions

In addition to standard precautions, further measures are followed when a patient may be infected with a pathogen or communicable disease. The type of precaution taken is indicated by posting the appropriate sign on the door (Figure 4-1).

The three levels of transmission-based precautions are as follows:

1. Use *airborne precautions* for diseases transported by the airborne route (see Table 4-1). Care providers use high-efficiency particulate air filter respirators (or other respirators that filter inspired air) for protection. In addition, a negative airflow ventilation system room is needed for tuberculosis. The patient in airborne precautions must wear a surgical mask when leaving the room to filter expired air. Label the patient's room with a sign instructing visitors to report to the nurse before entering (Figure 4-2).

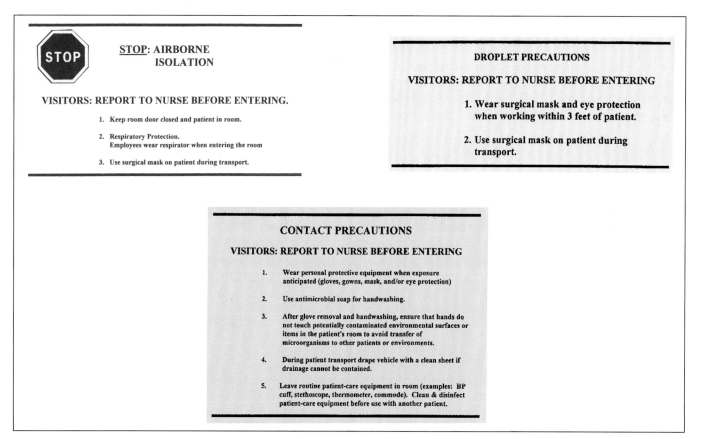

Figure 4-1 *Isolation signs.*

TABLE 4-1	Examples of Diseases Requiring Transmission-Based Precautions	
Airborne	**Droplet**	**Contact**
Measles	*Haemophilus influenzae* type b	Gastrointestinal illness (e.g.)
Varicella (chickenpox)	Rubella	*Clostridium difficile*
Tuberculosis	Pertussis	*E. coli*
	Mumps	*Hepatitis A*
	Pneumonia	Skin infections (e.g.)
		Scabies
		Impetigo
		Genital
		Herpes simplex
		Chlamydia
		Syphilis
		Gonorrhea

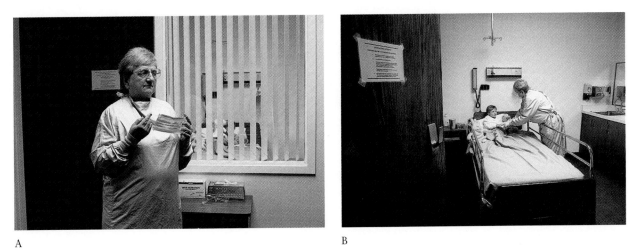

A   B

Figure 4-2 *For patients in airborne isolation, gowns and masks may be worn (A), and the door must be clearly labeled with a sign instructing visitors to stop at the nursing station before entering (B).*

2. Institute *droplet precautions* for diseases transmitted by the droplet route. A surgical mask is needed when coming within 3 feet of the patient. The patient wears a mask when leaving the room. The room door can remain open, and special respirators are not required.

   RATIONALE: *The large particle droplets of these diseases cannot travel over 3 feet.*

3. Use *contact precautions* for diseases that spread by direct contact with the skin or by indirect contact with a contaminated object in the patient's environment. Apply gloves for all care. Gowns are worn if the health care professional's clothing may come in contact with contaminated surfaces or the patient. Patients should be placed in a private room or with other patients with the same pathogen.

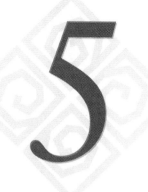

Physical Assessment

Chapter Outline

Growth Measurements

The accurate assessment of growth is important throughout childhood to assure one's health or to identify the impact of disease on the child. Growth charts for boys and girls are provided in Appendix A.

SKILL 5-1 Length

Until a child is 2 years of age, length is measured with the child in the supine position, even after the child is able to stand independently. The length measurement is the standard for accurate assessment of growth in children under 2 years of age. A difference in length and height measurements for children does exist. If height were plotted on a length-based growth chart, a true assessment of the child's growth over time could not be determined.

PREPARATION

1. Have the parent remove any hat or shoes the infant is wearing.

EQUIPMENT AND SUPPLIES

- Measuring board or other length-measuring device

PROCEDURE

1. When using a measuring board, place the infant's head against the top of the board.

2. Use the parent or an assistant to hold the infant's head in the midline and gently push down on the knees until the legs are straight.
   RATIONALE: *Because of the normally flexed posture of the infant, the body must be extended to obtain an accurate measurement.*

3. Position the heels of the feet on the footboard and record the length to the nearest 0.5 cm (0.25 in.). (Figure 5-1).

4. Repeat the measurement for accuracy. If a difference between the two readings is found, take the average reading for documentation.

5. Plot the measurement for the child's age on the standardized growth curve (see Appendix A).

If such a measuring device is not available, place the infant on a paper sheet. Make one mark at the vertex of the head and another at the heel. Then measure the distance between the two marks. Record the length in centimeters or inches.

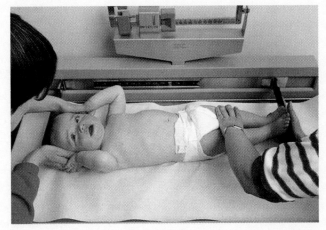

Figure 5-1 *Measuring an infant's length.*

SKILL 5-2 Height

After the age of 2 to 3 years, height is measured with the child standing upright against a wall with a stadiometer (Figure 5-2).

PREPARATION

1. Have the child remove the shoes and hat.

EQUIPMENT AND SUPPLIES

- Stadiometer or platform scale with stature-measuring device

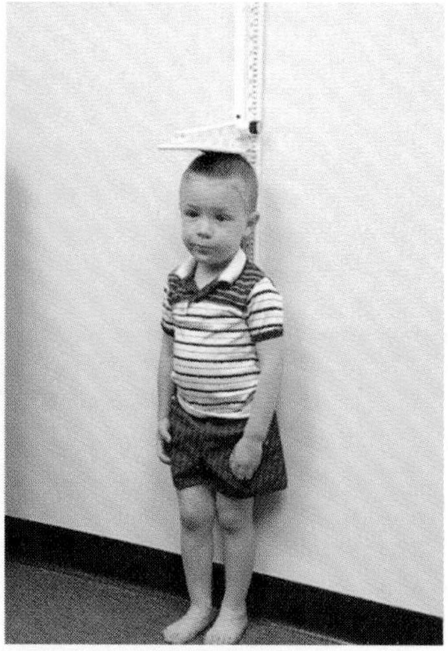

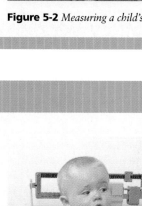

Figure 5-2 *Measuring a child's height.*

PROCEDURE

1. With shoes removed, have the child stand straight with the back to the wall. The head should be held erect and in the midline position.

2. The shoulders, buttocks, and heels should touch the wall. The outer canthus of the eyes should be on the same horizontal plane as the external auditory canals.

   RATIONALE: *Positioning the head properly helps ensure consistency in placement of the head piece on the crown of the head.*

3. Move the head piece down to touch the crown.

4. Make the height reading to the nearest 0.5 cm (0.25 in.).

5. Plot the measurement for the child's age on the standardized growth curve (see Appendix A).

In the older child and adolescent, height is often measured using a platform scale with an attached stature-measuring device. Have the child stand erect facing forward. Move the stature-measuring device to the top of the head. Have the child step off the scale and read the height in centimeters or inches.

SKILL 5-3 Weight

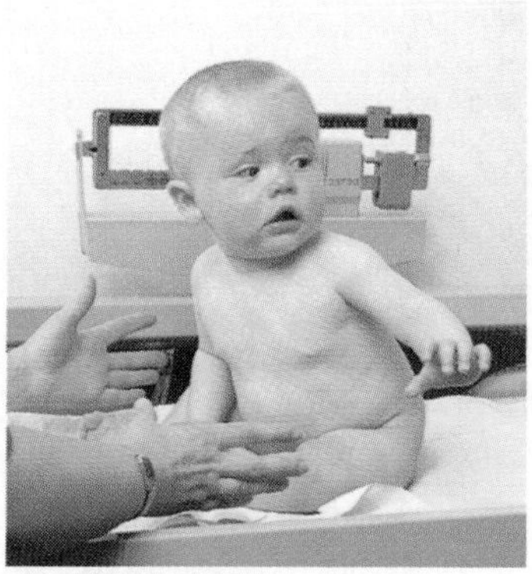

Infants are weighed on a platform scale (Figure 5-3), either in a supine or sitting position, depending on their age. Take care to ensure the infant's safety. Keep the room warm for comfort.

PREPARATION

1. Have the parent or assistant remove all of the infant's clothing and diaper. Weigh toddlers in their underclothes. Weigh older children in their street clothes with heavy clothing and shoes removed.

   RATIONALE: *It is important to try to minimize the amount of clothing worn by children when being weighed to improve comparisons with previous weights taken.*

2. Clean the infant scale tray between uses. Place a paper cover over the scale tray.

3. Check the balance of the scale before using it.

EQUIPMENT AND SUPPLIES

- Infant scale for infants
- Paper
- Standing scale for older children

Figure 5-3 *A platform scale is used to weigh an infant.*

PROCEDURE FOR INFANTS

1. Place the infant on the scale and keep a hand close.

   RATIONALE: *Infants move quickly and it is essential to protect the infant from falling.*

2. Distract the infant, and take the reading when the infant stops moving.

   RATIONALE: *It takes a few seconds of inactivity for the scale to settle on the infant's actual weight.*

3. Record the weight in the nearest 10 g (0.5 oz).

4. Plot the measurement for the child's age on the standardized growth curve (see Appendix A).

PROCEDURE FOR OLDER CHILDREN

The older child can be weighed on a standing scale.

1. Have the child stand still on the scale.

2. Move the weights until the scale is balanced for the child's weight.

3. Record the weight to the nearest 0.1 kg (0.25 lb).

4. Provide privacy for the older child and adolescent.

SKILL 5-4 Body Mass Index

The body mass index (BMI) uses a formula of kilograms per squared meter to assess nutritional status and total body weight relative to height. The child's BMI can be easily determined after plotting the length and weight or height and weight on the standardized growth curves (see Appendix A). For more detail, see Chapter 3 in *Pediatric Nursing, Caring for Children, Third Edition*.

> RATIONALE: *Tracking the change in BMI can often provide clues to nutritional problems, health promotion issues, or illness.*

SKILL 5-5 Head Circumference

Head circumference is usually measured at regular intervals until the child's second birthday.

PREPARATION

1. Remove any hat the infant is wearing.

EQUIPMENT AND SUPPLIES

- Disposable, nonstretching measuring tape with centimeter and millimeter markings

PROCEDURE

1. Wrap the tape around the head at the supraorbital prominence, above the ears, and around the occipital prominence (Figure 5-4). Take care to prevent a paper cut with the measuring tape.

   > RATIONALE: *This is usually the point of largest circumference of the head.*

2. Record the circumference in the nearest 0.5 cm (0.125 in.). Repeat the measurement to confirm the reading.

3. Plot the measurement for the child's age on the standardized growth curve (see Appendix A).

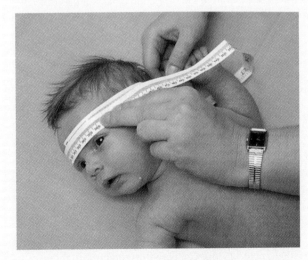

Figure 5-4 *Measuring head circumference.*

SKILL 5-6 Chest Circumference

Chest circumference may be measured until 1 year of age. The chest circumference measurement is a useful measurement in comparison with the head circumference when there is concern with the growth of either the head or chest.

PREPARATION

1. Remove all clothing from the child's chest.

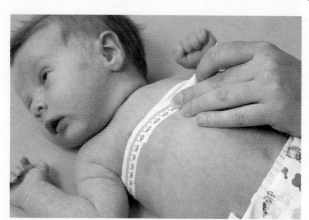

Figure 5-5 *Measuring chest circumference.*

EQUIPMENT AND SUPPLIES

- Disposable, nonstretching measuring tape with centimeter and millimeter markings

PROCEDURE

1. Wrap the tape measure around the chest, placed just under the axilla and at the nipple line (Figure 5-5).

2. Record the circumference measurement to the nearest 0.5 cm (0.125 in.).

3. Compare the chest circumference with the head circumference measurement.
   RATIONALE: *The head and chest circumferences will be approximately equal until after 1 year of age, when the chest circumference begins to surpass head circumference.*

SKILL 5-7 Abdominal Girth

Abdominal girth may occasionally be measured in children to monitor abdominal size that can vary with conditions such as edema from cardiac or renal disease.

PREPARATION

1. Remove all clothing from the abdomen.

EQUIPMENT AND SUPPLIES

- Disposable, nonstretching measuring tape with centimeter and millimeter markings

PROCEDURE

1. Wrap the tape around the abdomen at the level of the umbilicus, taking care to prevent a paper cut.

2. If the measurement is taken at another location on the abdomen, place ink marks at the location of the measurement.
   RATIONALE: *This action will enable you or another nurse to make a future measurement at the same location.*

3. Record the measurement to the nearest 0.5 cm (0.125 in.). Compare the reading with those taken previously to determine a change in size.

Vital Signs

Assessment of vital signs is also discussed in Chapter 4 of *Pediatric Nursing: Caring for Children, Third Edition.*

SKILL 5-8 Heart Rate

The procedure for assessing the heart rate is similar to that for adults; however, an apical heart rate is assessed in infants and young children.

PREPARATION

1. Move clothing away from the anterior chest.

2. Give the infant a pacifier or other distraction to get a resting pulse rate.

EQUIPMENT AND SUPPLIES

- Stethoscope

PROCEDURE

1. Place the stethoscope on the anterior chest at the fifth intercostal space in a midclavicular position (Figure 5-6).

   RATIONALE: *The apical heart rate is preferred in infants and young children, and is also used for older children when the condition warrants it. In infants and children, it is difficult to palpate the pulse in an extremity consistently enough to count the rate.*

2. Each "lub-dub" sound is one beat. Count the beats for 1 full minute, or for 30 seconds and multiply by 2.

3. While auscultating the heart rate, note if the rhythm is regular or irregular.

Pulse rates may be palpated in children over 3 years of age. Sites commonly used include the brachial, radial, femoral, and dorsal pedis. In addition, the pulse rhythm, strength, and amplitude may be checked.

- Note if the rhythm is regular or irregular.
- Compare the distal and proximal pulses in an extremity for strength.
- Record if the pulsation is normal, bounding, or thready.

The range of normal heart rates by age is listed in Table 5-1.

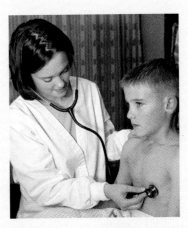

Figure 5-6 *Assessing the apical heart rate.*

TABLE 5-1	Normal Heart Rates for Children at Different Ages	
Age	Heart Rate Range (beats/min)	Average Heart Rate (beats/min)
Newborns	100–170	120
Infants to 2 years	80–130	110
2–6 years	70–120	100
6–10 years	70–110	90
10–16 years	60–100	85

SKILL 5-9 Respiratory Rate

The procedure for measuring a child's respiratory rate is essentially the same as for an adult; however, keep in mind the following points:

- Observe the abdomen rather than the chest rise and fall in an infant and young child.

  RATIONALE: *Because an infant's and young child's respirations are diaphragmatic, the abdomen moves more than the chest with breathing.*

- Abdominal movement in a child will be irregular.
- Count breaths for 1 full minute, or count for 30 seconds and multiply by 2.

The range of normal respiratory rates based on age is listed in Table 5-2.

TABLE 5-2	Normal Respiratory Rate Ranges for Each Age Group
Age	**Respiratory Rate per Minute**
Newborn	30–80
1 year	20–40
3 years	20–30
6 years	16–22
10 years	16–20
17 years	12–20

SKILL 5-10 Blood Pressure

The procedure for blood pressure measurement for the child is basically the same as for an adult. Whether manual or electronic equipment is being used, the correctly sized blood pressure cuff must be selected to obtain an accurate reading (Figure 5-7).

Figure 5-7 *Blood pressure cuffs are available in various types and sizes for pediatric patients.*

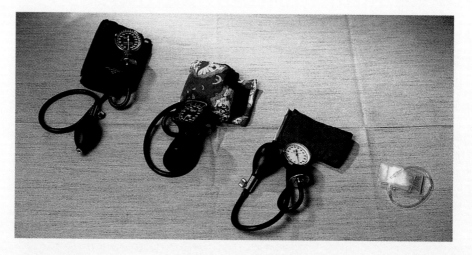

PREPARATION

1. To select the proper cuff size, compare the cuff with the size of the child's upper arm or thigh.
2. The bladder of the cuff should cover about 80% of the circumference of the extremity used.

3. The bladder width should cover about two-thirds of the upper arm or thigh.

   RATIONALE: *If the bladder is too small, the blood pressure reading will be falsely high; if it is too large, the pressure will be falsely low.*

EQUIPMENT AND SUPPLIES

- Various sizes of blood pressure cuffs
- Electronic blood pressure monitor
- Sphygomomanometer and stethoscope

PROCEDURE WITH DOPPLER ULTRASONOGRAPHY

Electronic equipment is often used to obtain the systolic blood pressure for infants and young children. With this technique, the frequency of ultrasonic waves is reflected by movement of the surface of the blood vessels, which differs slightly from that of other structures in the same area (Figure 5-8).

1. Place the cuff around the desired extremity.

2. Activate the equipment according to the manufacturer's recommendations.

3. Pressure is recorded as the number over "D."

PROCEDURE WITH MANUAL SPHYGOMOMANOMETER

1. Wrap the cuff snuggly around the desired extremity.

2. Palpate for the pulse, and place the stethoscope over the pulse area (Figure 5-9).

3. Close the air escape valve. Pump the cuff with the bulb until the gauge rises and no beat is auscultated. Continue pumping until the gauge rises another 20 to 30 mm.

4. Slowly release the air through the valve at 2 to 3 mm/sec while watching the falling gauge.

5. Note the number at which the first return of a pulse is heard; this is the systolic pressure.

6. Continue releasing the air to determine the diastolic pressure: If the child is less than 12 years, a muffled sound will be heard. Record this as the diastolic pressure. If the child is older than 12 years, all sound will disappear at the diastolic pressure.

7. Blood pressure is read as systolic over diastolic pressure (Table 5-3).

If the pulse cannot be auscultated, blood pressure can still be measured by palpation. Wrap the cuff around the desired extremity, close the air valve, and palpate for the pulse. Keeping your fingers on the pulse, pump the cuff with the bulb until the pulse is no longer felt. Slowly open the air valve, watching the gauge, and note the number at which the pulse is again palpated. This is the palpated systolic blood pressure read as the number over "P."

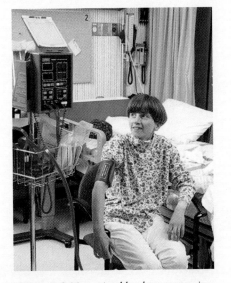

Figure 5-8 *Measuring blood pressure using Doppler ultrasonography.*

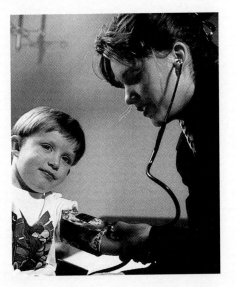

Figure 5-9 *Measuring blood pressure with a manual cuff.*

TABLE 5-3	Upper Limits (95th percentile) of Systolic and Diastolic Blood Pressure Values for Children of Different Ages by Selected Height Percentiles

Boys

	Systolic BP (mm Hg) by Height Percentile			Diastolic BP (mm Hg) by Height Percentile		
Age in Years	10th	50th	90th	10th	50th	90th
1	99	103	106	54	56	58
2	103	107	110	59	61	63
3	106	109	112	63	65	67
4	108	111	114	68	69	71
5	109	113	116	71	73	75
6	110	114	117	75	76	78
7	111	115	118	77	79	81
8	113	116	119	79	81	83
9	114	118	121	81	82	84
10	116	119	123	82	83	85
11	118	121	125	82	84	86
12	120	124	127	83	85	87
13	122	126	129	83	85	87
14	125	129	132	84	86	87
15	128	132	135	85	86	88
16	131	134	138	86	88	90
17	133	137	140	88	90	92

Girls

Age in Years	10th	50th	90th	10th	50th	90th
1	102	104	107	56	58	59
2	103	106	108	61	62	64
3	104	107	109	65	66	68
4	106	108	111	68	69	71
5	107	110	112	71	72	74
6	109	111	114	73	74	76
7	111	113	115	75	76	78
8	113	115	117	77	78	79
9	115	117	119	78	79	81
10	117	119	122	79	81	82
11	119	121	124	81	82	83
12	121	123	126	82	83	85
13	123	125	128	83	84	86
14	125	127	129	84	85	87
15	126	128	131	85	86	88
16	127	129	132	85	87	88
17	127	130	132	86	87	88

Note: Data from Rosner, B., Prineas, R.J., Loggie, J.M.H., & Daniels, S.R. (1993). Blood pressure nomograms for children and adolescents, by height, sex, and age, in the United States. *Journal of Pediatrics, 123,* 871–886.

Body Temperature

Body temperature can be measured in two scales: Fahrenheit or centigrade. Follow the manufacturer's guidelines for the use of electronic thermometers.

The four routes for measuring body temperature are tympanic, oral, axillary, and rectal.

SKILL 5-11 Tympanic Route

The tympanic route (Figure 5-10) is a convenient and fast method for taking temperatures in infants and children. Infrared technology provides a rapid reading. The ear temperature reflects the body temperature because the tympanic membrane shares its blood supply with the hypothalamus. The tympanic thermometer is easy to use and provides a rapid reading, and is noninvasive in nature. However, accurate measurement depends upon correct technique. (See Skill 2-8 for information on positioning a child for an ear exam.)

PREPARATION

1. Place the infant in a supine position on a flat surface. Stabilize the infant's head and turn the infant's head 90 degrees for easy access.

2. Position the child on parent's or assistant's lap with head secured.

EQUIPMENT AND SUPPLIES

- Tympanic thermometer with clean disposable probe

PROCEDURE: *Child Younger Than 1 Year*

1. If using the child's right ear, hold the thermometer in the right hand. For the child's left ear, hold the thermometer in the left hand.

2. Pull the pinna of the ear straight back and downward. Approach the ear from behind to direct the tip anteriorly to make sure the thermometer tip is aimed toward the tympanic membrane.
   RATIONALE: *The tip must be aimed at the tympanic membrane to ensure accuracy.*

3. Place the probe in the ear as far as possible to seal the canal. Turn on the scanner.

4. Leave the probe in the ear according to the manufacturer's recommendations.

5. Remove the probe, and read and record the temperature.

Child Older Than 1 Year

1. Pull the pinna up and back in children over about 3 years or up and downward under that age.

2. Place the probe and continue as described in step 1 for the child younger than 1 year.

3. Read and record the temperature.

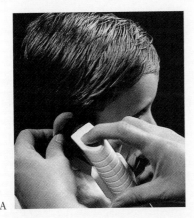
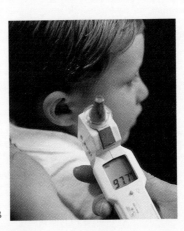

Figure 5-10 A, *Position for inserting thermometer when tympanic route is used.* **B,** *Digital readout of temperature appears within one minute.*

SKILL 5-12 Oral Route

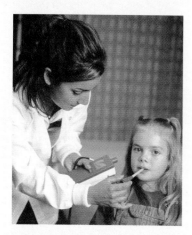

Fig. 5-11 *Measuring the oral temperature.*

The oral route may be used for the child over 3 years of age who is able to cooperate by holding the thermometer with the mouth closed.

PREPARATION

1. Assess the cooperation of the child to hold the thermometer in the mouth, under the tongue with the mouth closed.

EQUIPMENT AND SUPPLIES

- An electronic nonbreakable probe is preferred.

PROCEDURE

1. Place the oral probe or an electronic thermometer (with protective sheath) under the tongue and have the child enclose it with the lips (Figure 5-11).

2. Turn on the scanner and follow the manufacturer's recommendations. It will sound a tone or beep when finished. Remove the probe.

3. Read and record the temperature.

SKILL 5-13 Axillary Route

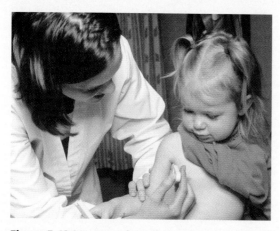

Figure 5-12 *Measuring the axillary temperature.*

The axillary route (Figure 5-12) is often used for newborns; children who are seizure prone, unconscious, or immunosuppressed; or who have a structural abnormality that precludes an alternate route. The axillary temperature is one degree lower than the oral temperature. Current research indicates that this method is not as accurate as other methods in identifying children with fevers.

PROCEDURE

- The electronic thermometer with protective sheath is held in place in the axilla, with the child's arm pressed close to the side.

- Turn on the scanner and follow the manufacturer's recommendations. It will sound a tone or beep when finished. Remove the probe.

- Read and record the temperature.

SKILL 5-14 Rectal Route

The rectal route should be used only when no other route is possible, due to the potential for rectal perforation and because most children view this as an intrusive procedure. The rectal temperature is one degree higher than the oral temperature.

PREPARATION

1. Place the infant or child prone on a bed or the parent's lap; turn the older child on the side.

EQUIPMENT AND SUPPLIES

- Electronic thermometer with sheath
- Water-soluble lubricant

PROCEDURE: *Clean Gloves*

1. Cover the tip of the electronic thermometer protective sheath with a water-soluble lubricant.

2. For the infant, place the tip 0.25 to 0.5 in. into the rectum. For the child, place the tip 1 in. into the rectum.

   RATIONALE: *This method reduces the risk of rectal perforation.*

3. Turn on the scanner and follow the manufacturer's recommendations. It will tone or beep when finished. Remove the probe.

4. Read and record the temperature.

Special Neurological Assessments

SKILL 5-15 Glasgow Coma Scale

The Glasgow Coma Scale is used to quantify the level of consciousness, thus enabling future comparison of improvement or deterioration in the child's condition. Pediatric criteria, which take into account the child's developmental age for each category of the test, have been established to assess responses to eye opening, verbal response, and motor response (Table 5-4).

TABLE 5-4		Glasgow Coma Scale for Assessment of Coma in Infants and Children	
Category	**Score**	**Infant and Young Child Criteria**	**Older Child and Adult Criteria**
Eye opening	4	Spontaneous opening	Spontaneous
	3	To loud noise	To verbal stimuli
	2	To pain	To pain
	1	No response	No response
Verbal response	5	Smiles, coos, cries to appropriate stimuli	Oriented to time, place, and person; uses appropriate words and phrases
	4	Irritable; cries	Confused
	3	Inappropriate crying	Inappropriate words or verbal response
	2	Grunts, moans	Incomprehensible words
	1	No response	No response
Motor response	6	Spontaneous movement	Obeys commands
	5	Withdraws to touch	Localizes pain
	4	Withdraws to pain	Withdraws to pain
	3	Abnormal flexion (decorticate)	Flexion to pain (decorticate)
	2	Abnormal extension (decerebrate)	Extention to pain (decerebrate)
	1	No response	No response

Add the score from each category to get the total. The maximum score is 15, indicating the best level of neurologic functioning. The minimum is 3, indicating total neurologic unresponsiveness.

Note: From Teasdale, G., & Jennett, B. (1974). Assessment of coma and impaired consciousness. Lancet, 2, 81–84; and James, H.E. (1986). Neurologic evaluation and support in the child with acute brain insult. *Pediatric Annals, 15(1),* 17.

PROCEDURE

1. When the child has had an injury to the head or has altered consciousness, assess each of the three categories of the Glasgow Coma Scale according to the criteria in the table.

2. Note the time and score for each category. Total the scores for all three categories to get the Glasgow Coma Score. A score of 15 is the maximum and indicates the best level of neurologic functioning.

3. Repeat the test at regular intervals.
   RATIONALE: *Since the test provides a numerical score for altered consciousness, regular measurements help detect subtle changes in the child's condition.*

4. Document the score and time performed.

SKILL 5-16 Neurovascular Assessment

A neurovascular assessment is performed frequently when an extremity is injured, such as from a fracture or circumferential burn. The circulatory status and nerve function are both evaluated in the injured extremity and compared with the other extremity. See Chapter 13 regarding cast care for application of this assessment.

PROCEDURE

1. Assess the swelling in the extremity associated with the injury.
   RATIONALE: *The swelling associated with the injury may constrict blood flow to the distal extremity and pinch the nerves.*

2. Assess the extremity distal to the injury for color and temperature and compare with the other extremity.

3. Assess the capillary refill time by pressing on a finger or toe for a couple of seconds, until the skin is blanched. Count how long it takes for blood or color to return to the area pressed. It should take 2 seconds or less.

4. Assess the extremity for pain and sensation (numbness, tingling, pins and needles sensation) and compare with the other extremity.

5. Consider all findings simultaneously to complete the neurovascular assessment.

6. Presence of most or all of the following indicates significantly impaired circulation and pressure or injury to the nerve that needs emergency intervention.
   - Pallor or cyanosis
   - Capillary refill time greater than 4 seconds
   - Cool or cold temperature
   - Moderate or severe pain
   - Numbness, tingling, or pins and needles sensation

7. Document the assessment, and repeat it frequently, especially if one or two findings are present.
   RATIONALE: *If the circulatory and neurologic constriction is not detected and promptly relieved, permanent damage to the distal extremity may result.*

COMMUNITY CONSIDERATIONS

Most states have laws regulating the ages or grades at which children must have vision screening performed, and what passing standards are accepted. Check your state laws or codes for guidelines.

Visual Acuity Screening

Vision acuity screening should begin at about 3 years of age, when the child can cooperate with the procedure. Several procedures may be used to screen visual acuity in children.

SKILL 5-17 Snellen Letter Chart

The Snellen letter (alphabet) chart (Figure 5-13A) is the most commonly used assessment tool for visual acuity. It consists of lines of letters in decreasing size.

- Most charts are designed for reading from a distance of 20 feet. When the child reads the line designated "20 feet" while standing 20 feet away, vision is 20/20. If, however, the child can only read the line labeled "40 feet" while standing 20 feet away, vision is 20/40.

- Charts are also available that can be used at a distance of 10 feet. A child who stands 10 feet from this chart and reads the 10-foot line (10/10) has vision equivalent to that of 20/20 when using the 20-foot chart.

SKILL 5-18 Snellen E or Picture Chart

For toddlers and children who have not yet mastered the alphabet, the Snellen E chart (Figure 5-13B) or picture chart (Figure 5-13c) may be used.

- On the E chart, the capital letter E is shown facing in different directions. The child is asked to point in the direction of the "legs" of the E. Another option is to give the child a paper with an E on it and have the child turn it in the direction the E is pointing on the chart.

- A variation of this test is the Blackbird Eye Test, in which a blackbird flies in a shape similar to an E. The child identifies which direction the bird is flying.

- The picture chart shows commonly identified silhouettes (e.g., house, apple, umbrella) lined up. The child is asked to identify the pictures.

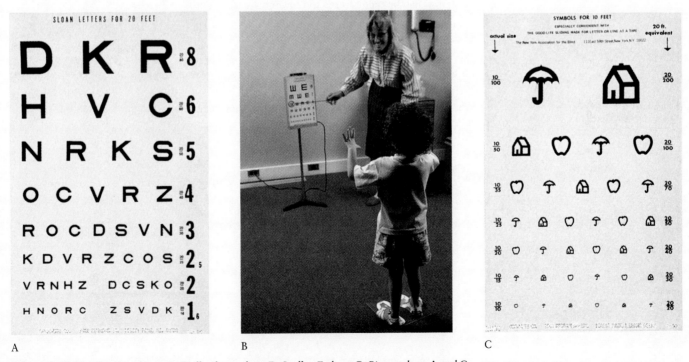

A   B   C

Figure 5-13 *Visual acuity charts.* **A,** *Snellen letter chart.* **B,** *Snellen E chart.* **C,** *Picture chart.* **A** *and* **C**
Courtesy of the *National Society to Prevent Blindness,* Shaumberg, IL.

SKILL 5-19 HOTV

For the HOTV eye test, the child looks at an HOTV chart positioned either 10 or 20 feet away and either names the letters or points to them on a card held close by. The procedure followed is the same as with the Snellen test, but because children can point to the letters on the chart in front of them, they do not need to know the alphabet. The HOTV test can also be used after a practice session with children who do not speak English.

PREPARATION

1. With the young child, make a game of identifying the direction of the E or the picture.
   RATIONALE: *This ensures that the child understands the directions for the test to improve the chances of an accurate screening test result.*

2. Place the chart at the child's eye level and in good lighting.

EQUIPMENT AND SUPPLIES

- Screening Chart
- Card or other item to cover one eye

PROCEDURE

1. Place the heels of the child at the 20-foot mark (or 10-foot mark if using that chart).

2. Assess each eye separately and then both together. If the child wears glasses, check the vision both with and without glasses. If the child is wearing contacts, leave them in and note that the results were with contacts.
   RATIONALE: *It is important to detect significant differences in visual acuity of the eyes of children under 5 years. When one eye has poorer vision than the other, the brain may decide to stop using the eye with poor vision, leading to further vision deterioration. Corrective lenses are required to enable the child to use both eyes and to preserve vision.*

3. While one eye is being tested, use the child's hand, a patch, or a piece of cardboard to cover the other eye. Tell the child to keep the covered eye open during the testing.

4. Observe for squinting, moving the head forward (to be closer to the chart), excessive blinking, or tearing during the examination.
   RATIONALE: *These signs may indicate a vision problem.*

5. Record the last line the child can read correctly (i.e., the last line in which the child reads more than half the symbols on the line). Refer to Table 5-5 for expected visual acuity by age.

6. When a child's vision is not within the passing standards range for age, the child should be retested in 1 to 2 weeks. If the results are still unsatisfactory, make the appropriate referral to the child's pediatrician or other health care provider, an ophthalmologist, or an optometrist.

TABLE 5-5	Passing Standards for Visual Acuity Testing Based on Age

Age	Visual Acuity
3–4 years	20/40
5 years	20/30
6 years	20/20

Hearing Acuity Screening

Hearing acuity screening is important to perform to ensure that the child is able to hear for speech and language development to occur. Newborn and infant hearing screening is performed using evoked otoacoustic emission and auditory brainstem response. See Chapter 19 of *Pediatric Nursing: Caring for Children, Third Edition*, for further description.

Several procedures may be used to screen hearing acuity in children. Various conditions during childhood, such as frequent ear infections, could result in a hearing loss.

SKILL 5-20 Pure Tone Audiometry

This procedure screens for hearing using air conduction. It is used on cooperative children over the age of 3 years. It can detect sensorineural hearing loss, but it does not detect fluid in the middle ear.

PREPARATION

1. Explain the procedure to the child. When screening a large group of children, such as in a school, the machine can be taken to the classroom for demonstration and practice.

2. Explain the procedure in terms the child can understand. Show the earphones. Turn the sound loud enough for the child to hear and practice raising a hand in response to the sound.
   RATIONALE: *This action helps ensure accurate results from the screening test.*

3. If a sound-proof room is not available, the audiometer should be set up in a quiet environment.
   RATIONALE: *It is important to reduce exposure to other sources of sound that could interfere with the child's response to the audiometer's sounds.*

4. Check the transmission of sound to be sure both ear phones work properly.

5. Clean the head phones with an alcohol swab between use.
   RATIONALE: *This practice removes most microorganisms for infection control between children.*

EQUIPMENT AND SUPPLIES

- Calibrated audiometer
- Scoring sheet
- Alcohol swabs

PROCEDURE

1. Position the child so that his or her back is toward the machine and faced away from the tester.
   RATIONALE: *This position ensures that the child cannot see the examiner press the lever to present the sound, and cannot receive visual cues from the examiner's face when the sound is presented.*

2. Place the headset on the child's head and adjust for a proper fit.

3. Follow directions for using the audiometer. Deliver sounds and watch for the child to raise a hand when heard. The sound cue is given to the child using a random order when testing the ears.
   RATIONALE: *This action ensures that the child cannot anticipate the sound and potentially cause an inaccurate interpretation of the screening test.*

4. Test each ear at the following pitches: 500, 1000, 2000, and 4000 Hz at increasing levels of loudness (decibels).

5. If the child does not pass the screening with both ears, retest the child in 2 weeks. If the child still does not pass, refer for further evaluation (Table 5-6).
   RATIONALE: *The child with an upper respiratory infection may not hear well and needs time for the infection to improve. Continued failure of the screening may indicate a hearing problem.*

COMMUNITY CONSIDERATIONS

Each state has specific laws mandating when children attending school should be screened for hearing acuity, and the hertz and decibel levels to be included. Consult your state school code for guidance about local requirements.

GROWTH AND DEVELOPMENT

If the young child does not seem to understand what to do once screening begins, remove the headphones and practice more. Have blocks ready and instruct the child to place a block in a basket when hearing the sound. Turn up the decibel level slightly and practice until the child understands. Then turn the decibel level back to the appropriate screening level.

CLINICAL TIP

The sounds of the audiometer are delivered at hertz levels, or the frequency of sound in cycles per second. Lower numbers indicate lower sounds, such as speech tones. Higher numbers indicate higher sounds, such as heard in music. The decibels, loudness of the sounds, can also be controlled by the audiometer.

TABLE 5-6	Passing Standards for Hearing Acuity with Pure Tone Audiometer
Hertz	**Decibels**
500	20–25
1000	20–25
2000	20–25
4000	25

SKILL 5-21 Tympanometry

Tympanometry provides an estimate of middle ear pressure and an indirect measure of tympanic membrane compliance (movement). Older infants and children can be tested. Abnormal findings often indicate fluid accumulation in the middle ear that prevents the efficient transmission of sound to the inner ear. This can result in hearing loss over time.

PREPARATION

Explain the procedure to the child and parents and the need for the child to hold still.

EQUIPMENT AND SUPPLIES

- Calibrated tympanometer
- Disposable ear piece
- Graph paper

PROCEDURE

1. Encourage the child to hold still during the test. The infant and young child may need assistance in holding still.

   RATIONALE: *Lack of movement reduces the chance of pain or injury from the ear piece in the auditory canal.*

2. Insert the ear piece with the tympanometer probe into the auditory canal until the canal is sealed and air tight.

   RATIONALE: *The canal must be sealed tight to get an accurate measurement of the pressure it takes to move the tympanic membrane.*

3. Turn on the tympanometer according to the manufacturer's instructions and emit the tone. The pressure is measured by the probe and plots it on a graph (Figure 5-14).

4. Repeat procedure in the other ear.

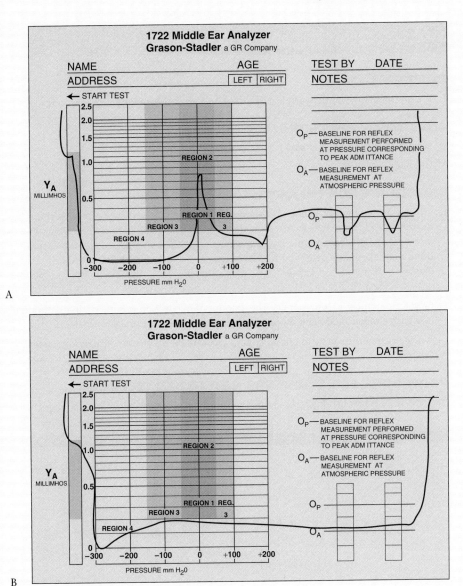

A

B

Figure 5-14 *A*, This tympanogram demonstrates normal hearing as evidenced by the curve showing the tympanic membrane's movement when a sound wave is emitted into the ear canal. Mobility is between 0.2 mL and 1.0 mL, the normal range. *B*, In contrast, note the flat pattern in the second tympanogram, which shows very restricted mobility of the tympanic membrane in response to sound.

Fluid and Electrolyte Balance: Intake and Output

Intake and output (I and O) is a measurement of fluid and electrolyte balance in the body. Input is measured as for adults, recording the fluids delivered to the child through parenteral or oral routes in cubic centimeters (cc) or milliliters (mL). See Chapter 11 of *Pediatric Nursing: Caring for Children, Third Edition,* for more details.

Output is a measurement of what is expelled, drained, secreted, or suctioned from the body. Output sources include urine, stool, vomitus, sweat, drainage from wounds, and nasogastric suction. Output for older children can be measured as for adults with a graduated cylinder, and recorded in cubic centimeters or milliliters.

Accurate measurement of I and O is documented for many children, such as those receiving intravenous fluids or certain medications; after major surgery; and those with serious infections, renal disease or kidney damage, congestive heart failure, diabetes mellitus, dehydration or hypovolemia, or severe thermal burns.

SKILL 5-22 Intake and Output Measurement

PREPARATION

1. Weigh the diapers to be worn by the infant and mark the weight in grams on the diapers.

EQUIPMENT AND SUPPLIES

- Scale with gram measurement
- Graduated cylinder

PROCEDURE FOR INFANTS: *Clean Gloves*

1. When a precise measurement of output is needed, weigh the diaper after the infant has voided or stooled. Disadvantages to this procedure include the inability to differentiate between urine and stool weights because the two substances may mix in the diaper, and the evaporation of urine that takes place after about 30 minutes.

   RATIONALE: *For each 1-g increase in weight of the diaper, 1 mL of liquid has been excreted by the infant.*

2. Count the number of wet diapers. The amount of micturition is fairly standard during infancy and early toddlerhood. Four to eight wet diapers per day is usually normal.

3. A urine bag may be used to obtain a fairly accurate measurement. Watch for any leakage. See Chapter 6.

PROCEDURE FOR TODDLERS AND OLDER CHILDREN

Once the child is toilet trained, the output is measured as for adults with a graduated cylinder.

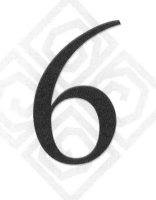

6

Specimen Collection

Chapter Outline

In the collection of any type of specimen, it is the nurse's responsibility to be sure that the specimen is collected accurately, labeled correctly, and sent to the laboratory using any special techniques needed such as immediate transport or maintaining on ice.

Blood Samples

The two methods of obtaining blood samples in children are capillary puncture and venipuncture.

A capillary puncture may be used to obtain a sample for complete blood count, reticulocyte count, platelet count, or blood chemistries such as electrolyte, glucose, or drug levels.

SKILL 6-1 Performing a Capillary Puncture

PREPARATION

1. Explain to the child and parents what will be done and what the child is likely to feel.

2. Have another nurse, an assistant, or the parent ready to restrain the child.

3. Choose the appropriate site. Puncture sites include the plantar surface of the heel (Figure 6-1) (for newborns and children under the age of 1 year), the great toe (for children over 1 year), and the palmar surface of the tip of the third or fourth finger.

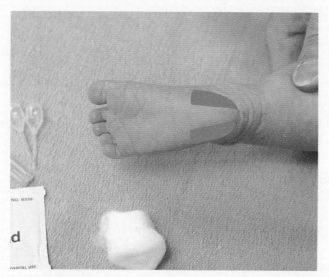

Figure 6-1 *Heel sites for capillary puncture.*

EQUIPMENT AND SUPPLIES

- Alcohol swabs
- Lancet
- Appropriate micro-size blood collection tubes

PROCEDURE: *Clean Gloves*

1. Apply gloves

2. *Finger stick.* Hold the child's hand with the nondominant hand (or have an assistant hold it), keeping the finger to be used extended and pointed down.

   Heel stick. Hold the child's foot in the nondominant hand, supporting the dorsum of the foot with the thumb and the child's ankle with the other fingers.

   Toe stick. Grasp the child's foot across the dorsum with the nondominant hand, supporting the child's toe with the thumb on the plantar surface.

3. Clean the site with alcohol.

4. Using the dominant hand, pierce the skin with the lancet.

5. Wipe the first drop of blood away with the gauze.
   RATIONALE: *The first drop may be contaminated by skin contact and the blood cells may have been traumatized during the stick.*

6. Using a milking motion, gently squeeze the site and direct the blood into the appropriate tube.

7. When collection is complete, have an assistant hold the gauze on the site until the bleeding has stopped. Apply an adhesive bandage.

SKILL 6-2 Newborn Screening

Blood screening of the neonate is performed to evaluate blood sugar and to assess for phenylketonuria, hypothryoidism, and other diseases. A small amount of blood can usually be obtained by heel stick for these tests.

PREPARATION

1. Examine newborn's record for results of any prior tests.
2. Verify test and procedures for present test.

EQUIPMENT AND SUPPLIES

- Lancet
- Capillary tube
- Metabolic screening card
- Washcloth rinsed in warm water (optional)

PROCEDURE: *Clean Gloves*

1. Wrap the warm washcloth gently around the foot for a few moments if desired.
   RATIONALE: *The warmth facilitates blood flow to the foot and ensures easy access to necessary blood for the test.*

2. Don gloves.

3. Flexing the infants forefoot up toward the leg (dorsiflexion), use the lancet to puncture the heel, collecting one large drop of blood.

4. The blood may be placed in a capillary tube, onto a metabolic screening card, or onto a glucose reagent strip, depending on the test desired.

5. To place blood on a screening card, completely fill the indicated circles (see Figure 6-2).

6. Allow the paper to air dry in horizontal position at room temperature on the screening form. Alternatively, if the blood is being sent to the laboratory in the capillary tube, seal the open end with Critoseal and transport according to agency policy.

7. Clearly label the blood samples and cards with the newborn's identifying information. Record the day and time, and the child's age in hours.
   RATIONALE: *Timing of certain tests is important in interpretation of results. Phenylketonuria testing must be done after 24 hours of age for accurate results, while metabolic screening is collected before 72 hours of age.*

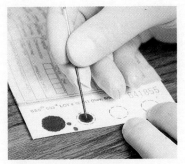

Figure 6-2 *Collecting a blood sample from the newborn for neonatal metabolic screening.*

COMMUNITY CONSIDERATIONS

When metabolic screening cards are completed in an office or clinic visit in the first days after birth, the specimen collected must be sent to the laboratory within 24 hours of collection.

SKILL 6-3 Blood Glucose Meters

Diabetic children commonly perform capillary punctures several times daily to measure their blood glucose with a small instrument.

PREPARATION: *Clean Gloves*

1. The procedure is explained to child and family.

2. The nurse demonstrates the procedure as needed and observes the child or family on return demonstration.

3. The diabetic child is taught over time how to safely perform repeated blood glucose tests and how to maintain materials.

EQUIPMENT AND SUPPLIES

- Reagent strips
- Blood glucose meter

Diabetic children who perform fingersticks for blood glucose analysis should be taught about safe practices for cleaning blood from surfaces by using bleach solution. Safe storage is needed to prevent young children from having access to the lancets. Identify a place in the school where the child can keep glucose-monitoring equipment and perform the procedure in private.

- Alcohol swab
- Lancet

PROCEDURE: *Clean Gloves*

1. Child and any assistants wash hands.
   RATIONALE: *This procedure removes surface contaminants to reduce chance of infection.*

2. Assistants wear gloves.

3. Clean finger to be used with alcohol if desired, but not necessary for diabetic with repeated tests (Figure 6-3).
   RATIONALE: *With repeated testing, alcohol can cause drying and cracking of the skin. Washing with soap and water removes most surface contaminants.*

4. Milk the finger gently or warm hand if cold.
   RATIONALE: *This practice encourages blood circulation to the fingertip so that the sample can be easily obtained.*

5. Quickly puncture the fingertip with the lancet.

6. Apply a drop of blood to the reagent strip.

7. Place the strip into the glucose meter and read instrument as instructed (Figure 6-4).

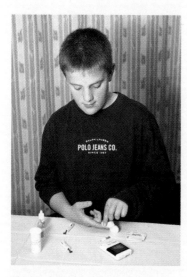

Figure 6-3 *The child is cleaning his finger prior to piercing the skin for blood glucose monitoring.*

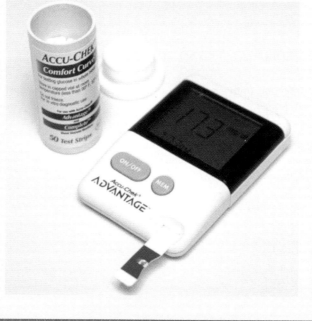

Figure 6-4 *Blood glucose monitors are small and quickly analyze a drop of blood and display the blood glucose in mg/dL.*

Venipuncture, or the puncturing of a vein, is used to obtain a sample for complete blood count, blood culture, sedimentation rate, blood type and crossmatch, blood clotting times, drug screen, ammonia level, or fibrinogen level.

SKILL 6-4 Performing a Venipuncture

PREPARATION

1. Choose the appropriate site. The veins of the antecubital fossa or forearm are usually the best choice because of their accessibility; however, the dorsum of the hand or foot also may be used. (Refer to page 68 of Chapter 8 for site location.)

EQUIPMENT AND SUPPLIES

- Tourniquet
- 20- to 27-gauge needle with attached syringe (slightly larger than volume of blood needed)
- Large-bore (19-gauge) needle
- Appropriate blood collection tubes

PROCEDURE: *Clean Gloves*

1. Apply gloves.

2. Place a tourniquet proximal to the desired vein to distend it. If necessary, hold the extremity below heart level, gently rub or tap the vein, or apply a warm compress to promote dilation of the vein (Figure 6–5A).

3. Locate the vein by inspection (wiping with alcohol will make the vein shine) or palpation.

4. Once the vein has been located, clean the skin with alcohol or povidone-iodine, using an outward circular motion (Figure 6-5B). Let dry.

5. With the nondominant hand, hold the skin taut, gently pulling with the thumb just under the site of the puncture.

6. Puncture the skin with the needle, beveled up at a 15-degree angle and directed toward the vein. When blood appears in the tube, gently pull back on the syringe (Figure 6-5C).

7. Release the tourniquet after all the blood has been collected. Remove the needle at the same angle used for entry and apply pressure to the site with gauze (alcohol will sting).

8. Have the assistant or parent maintain pressure for a few minutes until the bleeding has stopped, at which point an adhesive bandage can be placed. Meanwhile, remove the needle from the syringe and discard.

9. Attach the large-bore (19-gauge) needle, and expel blood into the appropriate collection tubes as soon as possible.

CLINICAL TIP—VENIPUNCTURE

- Make sure the tourniquet is tight enough to restrict venous but not arterial blood flow.

- Keep the bevel of the needle up.

- Do not draw back too hard or rapidly on the syringe because the vein will collapse.

- If blood fails to enter the syringe, the needle may not be placed correctly in the vein. Advance it slightly.

- If a flash was seen initially but blood no longer appears, the needle may be located incorrectly in the vein. Gently draw back on the needle slightly.

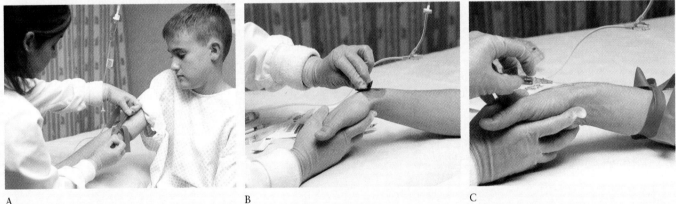

Figure 6-5 *Venipuncture procedure* **A,** *The tourniquet is applied to restrict venous blood flow.* **B,** *The area for venipuncture is cleaned by the nurse with betadine and alcohol solutions and dried with a cotton ball.* **C,** *The needle is placed with the bevel up and gently inserted into the identified vein.*

SKILL 6-5 Blood Cultures

Cultures of blood samples may be performed to determine if a child has septicemia. Such samples are commonly drawn two different times a few hours apart to assist in accurate diagnosis of causative microorganisms.

PREPARATION

1. Choose the appropriate site. The veins of the antecubital fossa or forearm are usually the best choice because of their accessibility. However, the dorsum of the hand or foot also may be used. (Refer to page 68 of Chapter 8 for site location.)

EQUIPMENT AND SUPPLIES

- Tourniquet
- 20- to 27-gauge needle with attached syringe (slightly larger than volume of blood needed)
- Large-bore (19-gauge) needle
- Appropriate blood collection tubes

PROCEDURE: *Sterile Gloves*

1. When infection is suspected, the first blood draws are done before starting antibiotics.
   RATIONALE: *Antibiotics may alter the results so that a microorganism is not detected.*

2. Apply sterile gloves, and thoroughly cleanse the skin with iodine and alcohol.
   RATIONALE: *Strict sterile technique reduces the chance that skin surface bacteria are found in the laboratory, leading to misdiagnosis.*

3. Use either venipuncture or an arterial line for samples as ordered.

4. Samples for the two different times are usually drawn from two different sites.
   RATIONALE: *Results can be compared to determine if microorganisms are present in the blood rather than just from skin contamination during the draw.*

5. Each blood draw specimen is placed in two different culture tubes—one for anaerobic and one for aerobic bacteria.

6. Carefully label and transport specimens as recommended by laboratory.

Urine Samples

A urine sample is obtained to assess for infection and to determine levels of blood, protein, glucose, acetone, bilirubin, drugs, hormones, metals, and electrolytes. Urine can also be evaluated for concentration/specific gravity, pH, and crystals or other substances.

A clean-catch urine specimen is needed to evaluate presence of microorganisms. The procedure varies according to the developmental level of the child. Infants and young children will have to be catheterized or can have a sterile urine bag placed. Older children can often void and provide a midstream voided specimen.

SKILL 6-6 Applying a Urine Collection Bag (Infant)

PREPARATION

1. Instruct parents about the procedure.

EQUIPMENT AND SUPPLIES

- Urine collection bag (newborn or pediatric size as needed)
- Soap solution, sterile water, and sterile cotton balls or packaged cleansing swabs for cleaning genitalia
- Sterile urine specimen container

PROCEDURE: *Clean Gloves*

1. Don gloves.

2. Remove the diaper and clean the skin well.

3. Remove gloves, wash hands, and apply new gloves. Wipe the genital area with a cotton ball and soap about three times (from the tip of the penis toward the scrotum for boys, and the clitoris toward the anus for girls). Repeat using sterile water and cotton balls to rinse. Use each cotton ball only once and discard. Alternately, about three packaged wipes can be used as described.

4. Attach the bag with the adhesive tabs (Figure 6-6): for girls, around the labia; for boys, around the scrotum.

5. Make sure the seal is tight to prevent leakage.

6. Check the bag frequently for urine.

To Remove a Bag Containing Urine—Sterile Gloves

7. Apply sterile gloves.

8. Gently pull the bag away from the skin. Fold the opening over and place the urine bag into the sterile specimen container.

9. Cap the container tightly.

10. Label with name, date, time, and send promptly to laboratory.

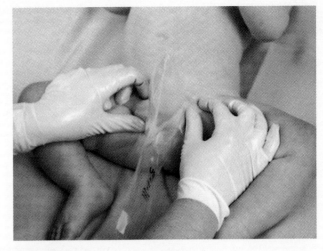

Figure 6-6 *Attaching the urine collection bag.*

SKILL 6-7 Collecting a Clean-Catch Urine Specimen (Older Child)

PREPARATION

1. Explain procedure to child and parent if present.

EQUIPMENT AND SUPPLIES

- Towelettes
- Sterile urine specimen container

PROCEDURE: *Clean Gloves*

Male

1. Instruct the older child to wash hands well, and then clean the head of his penis (after pulling back the foreskin, if not circumcised) three times, each time using a different towelette, moving from the urethral meatus outward.

2. Have the child urinate a small amount into the toilet, stop the flow, then urinate into the sterile container.

3. Cap the container tightly. Always wear gloves in case there are any urine spills on the container.

4. Label with name, date, time, and send promptly to laboratory.

Female

1. Instruct the older child to wash hands well, and then to sit back on the toilet as far as possible with legs apart. Have her spread her labia with her fingers and wipe each side with a separate towelette using a front-to-back stroke. Tell the child to use a third wipe to clean the meatus, repeating the front-to-back motion.

2. Have the child urinate a small amount into the toilet, stop the flow, then urinate into the sterile container.

3. Cap the container tightly. Wear gloves in case of any urine spills on the container.

4. Label with name, date, time, and send promptly to laboratory.

SKILL 6-8 Collecting a Catheter Specimen

PREPARATION

1. Explain procedure to child and parent if present.

EQUIPMENT AND SUPPLIES

- Clamp
- Alcohol swab
- Syringe with needle
- Sterile specimen container

PROCEDURE: *Clean Gloves*

1. Locate self-sealing port on urinary catheter tubing. The site is distal to the balloon that is in-serted to keep the catheter in place.

    RATIONALE: *Self-sealing rubber catheters have a port that can be accessed with a syringe. This technique cannot be performed on plastic or silicone catheters. The port is distal to the balloon to avoid puncturing and dislodging the catheter.*

2. Wash hands and apply gloves.

3. If there is no urine in the catheter apply clamp and wait for several minutes.

4. Clean port with alcohol swab.

    RATIONALE: *This cleaning minimizes the chance of transferring contami-nants from the catheter surface into the urinary tract.*

5. Insert needle on syringe into port at an angle. Release clamp if applied.

6. Withdraw urine and transfer to sterile specimen container. Discard syringe in sharps container.

7. Label with name, date, time, and send promptly to laboratory.

ROUTINE COLLECTION

When a sterile sample is not required, the same techniques may be used; how-ever, sterile gloves and technique while obtaining the sample are not needed. Clean gloves may be used to place urine bags or to clean the child prior to void-ing. A device may be placed on the toilet to collect the sample (Figure 6-7).

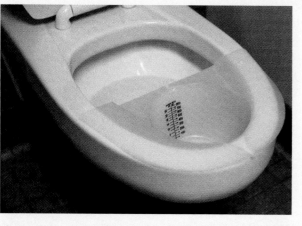

Figure 6-7 *A urine collection device for the toilet.*

Stool Culture

Stool cultures are used to detect the presence of bacteria and other organisms in the in-testinal tract. A sample for culture can be obtained from stool collected in a cup, from a diaper, or from a swab that has been gently inserted into the child's rectum. A test for parasites requires larger size samples and is usually submitted in a stool specimen cup-like container.

SKILL 6-9 Obtaining a Stool Specimen

PREPARATION

1. Gather supplies.

EQUIPMENT AND SUPPLIES

- Two culturette swabs or stool specimen container and two tongue blades

PROCEDURE: *Clean Gloves*

1. Don gloves.
2. Open one culturette swab, holding it in the dominant hand while keeping the cover in the nondominant hand.
3. Dip the swab into the stool. Replace the cover. Squeeze the bottom of the closed culturette to release the culture medium.
4. Repeat with the second culturette.
5. Label and promptly send to laboratory.

For Parasitic and Other Specimens

1. Don gloves.
2. Obtain specimen from diaper or container on toilet by using tongue blades.
3. Place specimen in stool container.
4. Remove gloves, label container, and send to laboratory.

Wound Culture

A culturette swab is used to obtain samples for microscopic examination from a wound or body site such as the eyes, ears, nose, throat, rectum, or vagina.

SKILL 6-10 Obtaining a Sample for Wound Culture

PREPARATION

1. Gather supplies.

EQUIPMENT AND SUPPLIES

- One culturette swab

PROCEDURE: *Sterile Gloves*

1. Don sterile gloves.
2. Open the culturette, holding it in the dominant hand while keeping the cover in the nondominant hand.
3. Gently swab the infected area.
4. Cover the swab and release the culture medium.
5. Label and promptly send to laboratory.

SKILL 6-11 Wound Irrigation

Wounds may be irrigated to clean away organisms and dead tissue and to promote healing. Irrigations may be done one time or repeated on a daily or more frequent basis.

PREPARATION: *Sterile Gloves*

1. Explain the procedure to the child and parent.

2. Perform a pain assessment.
   RATIONALE: *The child may need pain medication before the procedure begins to promote comfort.*

3. Place absorbent material under the area.

4. Apply sterile gloves and remove any dressings from the wound.

5. Observe type and amount of drainage for documentation after the procedure.

6. Discard gloves and wash hands.

EQUIPMENT AND SUPPLIES

- Irrigation solution as ordered
- Irrigation set or sterile syringes with irrigating tip
- Sterile basin
- Method for protecting bed
- Clean linens
- New topical medications and sterile dressing as ordered

PROCEDURE: *Sterile Gloves*

1. Check to be sure that pads and other absorbent materials are adequately situated under the area to be irrigated.

2. Set up sterile field and open supplies needed using sterile technique.

3. Apply sterile gloves.

4. Withdraw sterile solution for irrigation.
   RATIONALE: *Solutions are ordered for ability to clean the area or treat infection. Examples include isotonic saline, Ringers lactate, and dilute antibiotic solutions.*

5. Release solution from syringe, allowing it to flow over the wound. Collect in sterile basin under wound.

6. Repeat several times until solution is used and wound debris is cleansed.

7. Apply topical medications and dressing as ordered.

8. Clean and dry the child.

9. Once removing supplies, document observations of wound and the child's responses to the irrigation.
   RATIONALE: *The condition of the wound and the child's pain level may indicate healing and condition of the wound.*

Throat Culture

A culturette swab is used to obtain a sample from the throat for microscopic examination.

SKILL 6-12 Obtaining a Sample for a Throat Culture

PREPARATION

1. Gather supplies.

EQUIPMENT AND SUPPLIES

- Two culturette swabs
- Penlight

PROCEDURE: *Clean Gloves*

1. Don gloves.

2. Open the culturette, holding it in the dominant hand while keeping the cover in the nondominant hand.

3. Use the penlight as needed to provide adequate views of the throat.

4. Gently swab the back of the throat along each tonsillar area with a separate culturette.

5. Cover the swabs and release the culture medium.

6. Transfer promptly to the laboratory.

Respiratory Secretions

Secretions are obtained to detect bacteria that cause respiratory infections. Different techniques are used for infants and older children. The infant will need suctioning. The older child can cooperate and cough into the provided container.

SKILL 6-13 Collecting Respiratory Secretions from an Infant

PREPARATION

1. Gather supplies.

EQUIPMENT AND SUPPLIES

- Sterile suction catheter
- Sterile normal saline
- Suction trap

PROCEDURE: *Sterile Gloves*

1. According to the manufacturer's guidelines, attach the suction trap to low wall suction (60 mm Hg).

2. Apply gloves.

3. Suction the child's nose (refer to the description of suctioning in Chapter 10), using a small amount of sterile normal saline to clear the tubing.

4. Close the trap.

Note: This will provide a specimen from the nasopharyngeal area. If a tracheal specimen is needed, the deep suctioning technique described in Unit 9 should be consulted.

SKILL 6-14 Collecting Respiratory Secretions from a Child

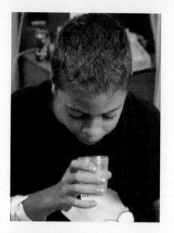

Figure 6-8 *Child supplying a sputum specimen.*

PREPARATION

1. Gather supplies.

EQUIPMENT AND SUPPLIES

- Sterile specimen container

PROCEDURE: *Clean Gloves*

1. Don gloves.

2. Encourage the child to take several deep breaths, then cough sputum up and spit it directly into the cup (Figure 6-8).

3. Close the cup.

Administration of Medication

Chapter Outline

Administration of Medication

Administering medications to children presents a number of challenges: deciding which drug forms to use, determining dosages, choosing methods and sites, and taking into account implications based on the child's development. See Table 7-1 for considerations needed when administering medications to children by various routes.

TABLE 7-1	Variations in Medication Administration to Children	
Route	**Developmental Consideration**	**Techniques**
Oral	Children under 5 years cannot generally swallow pills and capsules	▪ Medications are usually given in liquid form (e.g., elixir, syrup or suspension). ▪ Sometimes tablets are crushed or capsules are opened and mixed with one spoon of food. Check with pharmacy to be sure this does not inactivate the drug. Never crush enteric-coated or timed-release medicine. ▪ When choosing a vehicle for crushed tablets, use only one spoonful of applesauce, pudding, jelly, or similar food. ▪ Use TB syringe for amounts less that 1 mL to increase accuracy.
	Children may not want to take medicine.	▪ Position young children upright to avoid choking and aspiration. ▪ Give liquid medicines slowly by oral syringe (for infants) aimed at the inside of the cheek or by medicine cup (for toddler and preschooler) for drinking. ▪ Have the expectation that the medicine will be taken. Let children choose the type of fluid to drink after but do not ask if they will take their medicine now.
Rectal	Colon is small in size.	▪ For children under 3 years, the nurse's gloved fifth finger is used for insertion. After this age the index finger can usually be used. ▪ Lubricate the tip of the suppository.
Ophthalmic and Otic	Young children may be fearful of medicines placed in the eyes or ears.	▪ Adequate restraint is needed to avoid injury. ▪ The nurse's hand can be stabilized by resting the wrist on the child's head. ▪ Explanations and therapeutic play can be used with children old enough to explain the process of administration. ▪ Have medication at room temperature.
Topical	Skin of infants is thin and fragile.	▪ Only prescribed doses and medicines appropriate for young children should be used on the skin. ▪ Covering the area or keeping the child's hands occupied may be necessary to ensure adequate contact of medication with the skin.
Intramuscular	Anatomy and physiology of children differs from that of adults.	▪ Gluteus maximus muscle (dorsal gluteal site) must not be used until the child has been walking for at least 1 year. ▪ Vastus lateralis site is preferred for young children. ▪ Amounts to be administered should be limited to no more than 1–2 mL for ventrogluteal site depending on muscle size. ▪ The deltoid muscle is rarely used in young children except for the small amounts injected in some vaccines.
Intravenous	Veins are small and fragile.	▪ Careful maintenance of sites is needed. ▪ Common infusion sites include hands and feet, although scalp veins are sometimes used in infants.
	Fluid balance is critical.	▪ Infusion pumps require frequent monitoring. ▪ Syringe pumps are often used when minimal fluid is to be given over an extended period of time. ▪ Central lines are commonly used for long-term intravenous medication therapy.

Although the drug and the dosage are determined by the prescriber, it is imperative that the nurse observe the "five rights" of medication administration before any medication is given (Table 7-2).

Preparation

- Explain all procedures or treatments to the child and parents, based on the child's developmental stage and the level of understanding of both parties.

- Answer all questions before giving the medication.

- Identify any known drug allergies.

Documentation

- Once a medication is given, record the name of the drug, the route, the date and time, and, if appropriate, the site.

- Record the response to the medication, including desired effects and undesired side effects.

  RATIONALE: *A record of response is especially important with medications for pain control and those for treatment of an acute problem such as respiratory difficulty.*

Calculation

It is the nurse's responsibility to calculate the dosage of the medication ordered to determine if the dosage is within the normal range for the child's height and weight.

Dosages can be calculated using the child's weight (written as mg/kg) or total body surface area. This is determined by plotting the child's height and weight on a nomogram (see Appendix B). Draw a line connecting the two columns and note the results at the point where the drawn lines cross the center column. The dosage is ordered as mg/m^2.

TABLE 7-2	"Five Rights" of Medication Administration

1. Right medication
   - Compare the name of the drug on the medication sheet with the name of the drug on the label of the drug container three times. Check the container's expiration date.
   - Know the action of the drug.
   - Identify the potential side effects of the drug.
   - Use the pharmacy, hospital, or other drug formulary as a reference for medications with which you are unfamiliar.

2. Right patient
   - Verify the name on the medication sheet against the name on the child's identification band. When in a setting with no name band (e.g., clinic), verify the child's name with the child and parent by asking them to state the name.

3. Right time
   - When ordered for a specific time, a medication should be given within 20–30 minutes of that time.
   - For prn medications, check the last time the dose was given as well as the total 24-hour dose the child has received to verify that the child can receive another dose at this time.

4. Right route of administration
   - Always use the ordered route for administration of a medication. If a change is needed (such as a change from oral medication when a child is vomiting), check with the prescriber to get an order for a change in route.

5. Right dose
   - Calculate the ordered dose based on the child's weight in kilograms.
   - If in doubt about what constitutes an appropriate dose, compare with the pharmacy, hospital, or other drug formulary guidelines for recommended dose.
   - Question the order if the dose is outside of recommended amounts.

Example 1

The physician orders morphine (available as 10 mg/mL) for a 3-year-old child who weighs 15 kg. The recommended dose for children is 0.1 mg/kg. What dose is appropriate for the child's weight? How much volume should be drawn?

Answer

Recommended dose × Weight = Dose for patient
0.1 mg/kg × 15 kg = 1.5 mg
Dose desired/Dose on hand × Quantity in mL = Volume to be administered
1.5 mg/10 mg × 1 mL = 0.15 mL to be administered

Example 2

The physician orders phenobarbital (available as 65 mg/mL) for a 5-year-old child who weighs 20 kg. The recommended loading dose for the child is 10 to 20 mg/kg. The physician orders 250 mg to be infused over 30 minutes. Is this dose appropriate for the child's weight? How much volume should be drawn? How do you set the infusion pump?

Answer

Recommended dose × Weight = Desired dose
10 mg/kg × 20 kg = 200 mg
20 mg/kg × 20 kg = 400 mg
Dose of 250 mg is within recommended range.
Dose desired/dose on hand × Quantity in mL = Volume to be administered
250 mg/65 mg × 1 mL = 3.85 mL

Pump set up

The nurse determines the volume for the setup is 50 mL.
50 mL/30 min × 60 min/1 hr = mL/hr = 100 mL/hr
Rate = 100 mL/hr

Oral Medication

Children younger than 5 years of age usually have difficulty swallowing tablets and capsules. For this reason, most medications for pediatric use are also available in the form of elixirs, syrups, or suspensions. If a medication is only available in tablet or capsule form, it may need to be crushed before being administered. Be sure not to crush medications with enteric coating. Remember to wear clean gloves if your hands might come in contact with the child's saliva.

SKILL 7-1 Administering an Oral Medication

PREPARATION

1. Measure the medication accurately to ensure that the dose is correct.

2. If the oral medication is liquid (especially if less than 5 mL), it should be measured in a syringe or calibrated small medicine cup or dropper (Figure 7-1). A specially designed medication bottle may also be used.

3. If a tablet or pill needs to be crushed, place it in a mortar or between two paper medicine cups and crush it with a pestle. Once the tablet or pill has been pulverized, mix the powdered medication with a small amount of flavored substance such as juice, applesauce, or jelly to disguise any unpleasant flavor.

EQUIPMENT AND SUPPLIES

- Medicine cup, syringe, or other device for administering medication
- Medication

Figure 7-1 *Oral medications can be administered with various types of equipment, depending on the child's age.*

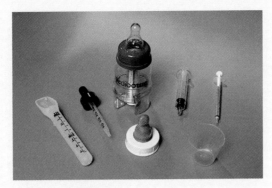

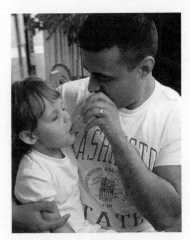

Figure 7-2 *This father needs to administer a medication to his daughter at home. He has been instructed how to hold her and administer the dose safely and effectively.*

PROCEDURE: *Clean Gloves*

Infant

1. A syringe or dropper provides the best control.

2. Apply gloves if needed.

3. Place small amounts of liquid along the side of the infant's mouth. Wait for the infant to swallow before giving more.

   RATIONALE: *This method helps to prevent aspiration and maximizes the chance that the infant will get all the medicine rather than spitting some out.*
   Alternative method: Have the infant suck the liquid through a nipple.

TODDLER OR YOUNG CHILD

1. Place the child firmly on the lap or the parent's lap in a sitting or modified supine position (Figure 7-2).

2. Apply gloves if needed.

3. Administer the medication slowly with a syringe or small medicine cup.

Intramuscular Injection

The site of the intramuscular injection (Figure 7-3) depends on the age of the child, the amount of muscle mass, and the density and volume of medication to be administered. Young infants may not tolerate volumes greater than 0.5 mL in a single site, whereas older infants or small children may be able to tolerate 1 mL per site. As the child grows, greater volumes can be administered. **Note:** The larger the volume of medication, the larger the muscle to be used. If possible, avoid areas that involve major blood vessels or nerves.

The preferred site for the infant is the vastus lateralis muscle (Figure 7-4), which lies along the midanterior lateral aspect of the thigh. After the child has been walking for 1 year, the dorsogluteal site can be used. However, because these muscles are poorly developed, they are not the ideal choice for a child less than 5 years old.

For the older child and adolescent, the sites are the same as for the adult: the vastus lateralis, deltoid, and ventrogluteal muscles.

Safety during all injections is challenging and important with children. Facilities are mandated to maintain a record of and annually review any injuries obtained by needle stick, and to evaluate and use safer medical devices. This helps to ensure safety for children and nurses (U.S. Occupational Safety and Health Administration, 2001).

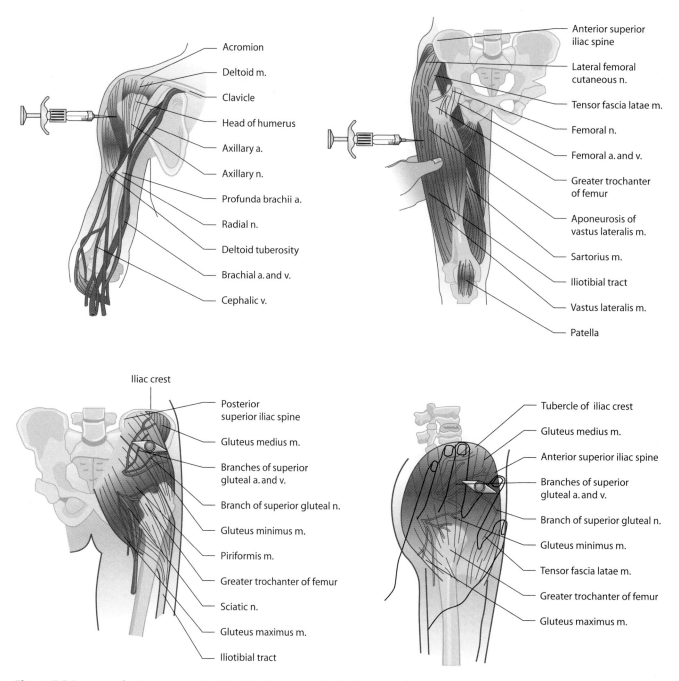

Figure label callouts:

Panel A (Deltoid):
- Acromion
- Deltoid m.
- Clavicle
- Head of humerus
- Axillary a.
- Axillary n.
- Profunda brachii a.
- Radial n.
- Deltoid tuberosity
- Brachial a. and v.
- Cephalic v.

Panel B (Vastus lateralis):
- Anterior superior iliac spine
- Lateral femoral cutaneous n.
- Tensor fascia latae m.
- Femoral n.
- Femoral a. and v.
- Greater trochanter of femur
- Aponeurosis of vastus lateralis m.
- Sartorius m.
- Iliotibial tract
- Vastus lateralis m.
- Patella

Panel C (Dorsogluteal):
- Iliac crest
- Posterior superior iliac spine
- Gluteus medius m.
- Branches of superior gluteal a. and v.
- Branch of superior gluteal n.
- Gluteus minimus m.
- Piriformis m.
- Greater trochanter of femur
- Sciatic n.
- Gluteus maximus m.
- Iliotibial tract

Panel D (Ventrogluteal):
- Tubercle of iliac crest
- Gluteus medius m.
- Anterior superior iliac spine
- Branches of superior gluteal a. and v.
- Branch of superior gluteal n.
- Gluteus minimus m.
- Tensor fascia latae m.
- Greater trochanter of femur
- Gluteus maximus m.

Figure 7-3 *Intramuscular injection sites. **A,** Deltoid. **B,** Vastus lateralis. **C,** Dorsogluteal. **D,** Ventrogluteal.*
Note: Redrawn and modified from Bindler, R., & Howry, L. (1997). *Pediatric drugs and nursing implications* (2nd ed., pp. 39–42). Stamford, CT: Appleton & Lange.

Figure 7-4 *In infants, the vastus lateralis muscle is preferred for intramuscular injections.*

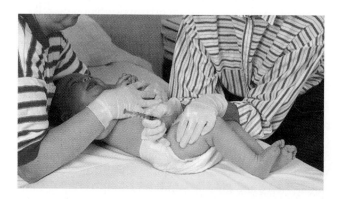

SKILL 7-2 Administering an Intramuscular Injection

PREPARATION

1. Select the syringe size according to the volume and dose of medication to be delivered. The needle must be long enough to penetrate the subcutaneous tissue and enter the muscle. Needles with a length of 0.5 to 1 in. (25 to 21 gauge) are recommended for infants and children.

2. Choose the appropriate site (see the preceding discussion).

EQUIPMENT AND SUPPLIES

- Syringe filled with medication
- Alcohol swab
- Gauze pad or cotton ball
- Small band-aid

PROCEDURE: *Clean Gloves*

1. Have another nurse, an assistant, or the parent restrain the child during the injection (Figure 7-5).
   RATIONALE: *Adequate restraint allows the procedure to be done safely and quickly and thereby minimize trauma for the child.*

2. Don gloves.

3. Locate the site. Clean with alcohol using an outward circular motion.

4. Grasp the muscle between the thumb and fingers for stabilization.

5. Remove the cap from the syringe. Insert the needle quickly at a 90-degree angle. Pull back the plunger.
   RATIONALE: *The 90-degree angle ensures entry into the muscle when the needle length is adequate. Pulling back on the plunger helps to rule out placement in a blood vessel.*

6. If no blood is aspirated, inject the medication, withdraw the needle, massage the area with a gauze pad or cotton ball (alcohol will sting), and return the child to a position of comfort. Apply a small band-aid if there is a drop of blood visible.

7. Do not recap the needle. Discard it in a puncture-resistant container according to standard precaution recommendations.

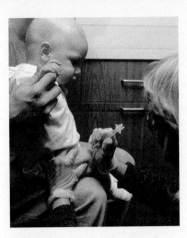

Figure 7-5 *The infant's legs and arms are controlled by the father and nurse so an injection can be administered safely.*

GROWTH AND DEVELOPMENT

Consider the child's age and developmental level when preparing for IM injections. Infants and toddlers will need to be held securely with only minimal explanations understood. The preschooler and young school-age child can often understand the reason for the injection. Explain what it will feel like, such as "I am going to clean your arm now with alcohol. This feels cold but does not hurt." And then, "You will feel the stick now and it's ok to tell me if it hurts." Children also can benefit from distractions that help them to manage the injection. "When I give the shot, let's count to ten together. Ok, it's in—one, two, three . . ." And finally, praise children for some part of their behavior. "I know you were scared but you held very still so we could do it fast."

Subcutaneous Injection

The site of the subcutaneous injection depends on the age of the child. Usually the dorsum of the upper arm or the anterior thigh is used in newborns, infants, and toddlers.

SKILL 7-3 Administering a Subcutaneous Injection

PREPARATION

1. Select the syringe size based on the volume or dose of medication to be delivered. The needle must be just long enough to penetrate the subcutaneous tissue, which lies below the skin and fat surface and above the muscle. Needles with a length of 3/8 to 5/8 in. (26 to 25 gauge) are recommended for infants and children.

2. Choose the appropriate site (see the preceding discussion).

EQUIPMENT AND SUPPLIES

- Syringe filled with medication
- Alcohol swab

- Gauze pad or cotton ball
- Small band-aid

PROCEDURE: *Clean Gloves*

1. Have another nurse, an assistant, or the parent restrain the child while the injection is being given.
2. Don gloves.
3. Locate the site. Clean with alcohol using an outward circular motion.
4. Pinch the skin between the thumb and index finger.
5. Remove the cap from the syringe. Insert the needle quickly at about a 45-degree angle. Release the skin and pull back the plunger.
   RATIONALE: *Use a 45-degree angle to inject into the subcutaneous tissue rather than into the underlying muscle.*
6. If no blood is aspirated, inject the medication, withdraw the needle at the angle at which it was inserted, massage the area with a gauze pad or cotton ball (alcohol will sting), and return the child to a position of comfort. Apply band-aid if there is a drop of blood present.
7. Do not recap the needle. Discard it in a puncture-resistant container according to standard precaution recommendations.

Intravenous Medication

The principles of intravenous medication administration in children are the same as those in adults. Special considerations when administering IV medication are discussed in this section. See Chapter 8 for accessing lines when a medication lock is in place or a central line is used.

Many drugs have specific dilution recommendations. Some medications are compatible with only specific fluids such as normal saline. Other medications must be given very slowly. Still other drugs can be administered quickly. Know your institutional or pharmacy standards for IV push or bolus administration (less than 10 minutes) versus intermittent medication administration. Be sure you know which medications are incompatible with one another and with types of intravenous fluids.

Special Considerations

It is recommended that IV medications for infants and children be put in a volume control chamber such as a Soluset or Metriset with the diluent and placed on an electronic pump for accurate administration. Alternatively, a syringe pump may be used, especially when fluid intake is closely regulated. Set the pump to the volume to be infused and the rate of infusion. Flush the line after the infusion to ensure that all medication has been administered, as some medication will remain in the distal tubing.

SKILL 7-4 Administering an Intravenous Medication

PREPARATION

1. Review the medication, administration recommendations, and the child's former responses and drug allergies.
2. Assess the IV line for patency.
3. If you are administering narcotics or benzodiazepines, have antagonists and ventilation equipment at bedside.
   RATIONALE: *The effect of most IV medications is almost immediate.*

4. Prepare the drug as needed. Reconstitution or withdrawal of solution from a vial or ampule may be needed.

EQUIPMENT AND SUPPLIES

- Syringe and needle or needleless system
- Prepared medication
- Dilution solutions
- Alcohol swabs

PROCEDURE: *Clean or Sterile Gloves*

1. Identify the child and explain procedure.

2. Assess intravenous line for patency and side effects. If the child has a medication lock in place, flush the line with 2–5 mL normal saline to check for patency or insert the IV line and allow to run for several minutes. Check the site again. See Chapter 8 for further detail.

3. Identify port on IV line to be used for push medications or for insertion of syringe pump. Generally a port proximal to the child is used, especially for intermittent infusion.
   RATIONALE: *A proximal port ensures that the medication will be delivered at the time administered. When an intravenous line is running slowly, it may take some time for the medication to travel from a distal port into the child.*

4. Identify medication port on volume control chamber for intermittent infusion.

5. Don gloves.

6. Clean the port and surrounding tubing with alcohol swab.
   RATIONALE: *Cleansing minimizes chance of instilling harmful organisms into the intravenous line.*

7. Insert needle or needleless syringe for IV push medication. While watching the time, slowly insert the medication in the ordered time frame. Observe the child carefully during administration. Stop the infusion if the child suddenly becomes lethargic or hyperactive or has other rapid change of behavior.
   RATIONALE: *Because IV push medications travel quickly into the vein, the appearance of side effects can occur rapidly. Close observation is needed to prevent undesired effects.*

8. When using a syringe pump, insert the primed tubing into a port close to the child. Set the infusion time as ordered for the medication.

9. When using intermittent medication administration, insert the medication in the proper dilution in the volume control chamber. Regulate the pump to administer the medication in the desired time.
   RATIONALE: *Medications should be administered in recommended time frames to ensure safety and effectiveness. Most antibiotics are administered over 30–60 minutes.*

10. Check on the child's condition several times during administration.
    RATIONALE: *Monitoring ensures that the child with side effects is identified and that the IV infusion is patent and running on time.*

11. At the end of administration, flush tubing with normal saline or running IV fluid.
    RATIONALE: *Flushing ensures that the entire amount of medication is infused and not left in the tubing. Flushing also removes medication from the line so that it will not mix with other drugs administered.*

12. Document administration and effects observed. Assess the IV line.

SAFETY PRECAUTIONS

It is recommended that needleless systems be used when available, to decrease the chance of needlestick injuries to patients and health care providers.

SAFETY PRECAUTIONS

It is important that tubing for IV administration and tubing and syringes for IV medication administration contain no air. Prime tubing properly to prevent air from being injected into the child's vein, which could be harmful.

Ophthalmic Medication

Young children fear having anything placed in their eyes, and special care is often needed to reduce the child's anxiety and promote cooperation during instillation of ophthalmic medications. An explanation of the procedure may help gain the child's cooperation. To prevent the transfer of pathogens to the eye, the medication and its dispensing port must be kept sterile.

SKILL 7-5 Administering an Ophthalmic Medication

HOME CARE CONSIDERATIONS: INSTILLING EYE MEDICATIONS

It can be challenging to safely instill eye medication into young children. Give parents the following suggestions.

- Wash hands well.

- Be sure the medicine is warmed to at least room temperature.

- Remove any drainage from the eye with a clean or sterile moist, warm cloth or gauze.

- Wash hands again.

- Have the child lying on the back with eyes closed.

- Gently pull the lower lid down to form a small pocket.

- Apply a thin string (for ointment) or drops of the medicine.

- Allow the eyelid to return to normal position.

- Have the child keep the eye closed for several seconds.

- Help prevent spread of the infection by keeping the child's hands clean.

- Enhance comfort by keeping the head elevated to decrease swelling and avoiding exposure to bright light.

PREPARATION

1. Gather supplies.

EQUIPMENT AND SUPPLIES

- Medication
- Sterile gloves

PROCEDURE: *Sterile Gloves*

1. Have another nurse, an assistant, or the parent restrain the child in a supine position with the child's head extended.

2. Don gloves.

3. Use the nondominant hand to pull the child's lower lid down while the other hand rests on the child's head (Figure 7-6).

4. Instill the drops or ointment into the conjunctival sac that has formed. *Alternative method:* Pull the lower lid out far enough to form a reservoir in which the medication can be instilled.

5. After the medication has been instilled, close the child's eyelids to prevent leakage.

6. Have the child lie quietly for a minimum of 30 seconds. Discourage the child from squeezing the eyes shut.

7. Dry the inner canthus of the eye.

8. Keep the child's head in the midline position to prevent the medication from contaminating the other eye.

9. When the child needs ophthalmic medication at home, instruct parents in proper technique.

Figure 7-6 *Administering an ophthalmic medication. The child is instructed to close his eyes and pretend to look up toward his head. The nurse then gently retracts the lower lid and inserts the medication.*

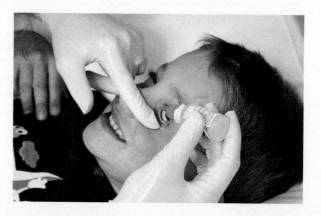

Contact Lens Care

Follow the prescriber's and family's directions for care of contact lenses. Encourage child and family to care for lenses when possible. General guidelines are as follows:

- Keep the lenses in the eyes for the recommended time only.

- Store each lens in the right or left containers as labeled.

- Wash hands carefully before contact with the child's eyes or lenses.

- Use a cleaning solution on the lens after its removal.

- Rinse the lens with the recommended rinsing solution.
- Keep the lenses in the case with the disinfecting storage solution.
- Note on the chart that the child wears lenses.

Eye Irrigation

Irrigation of the eye is performed to flush out a foreign body or a chemical irritant (Figure 7-7). Children often close the injured eye tightly, so getting them to relax for this procedure is important. Care must be taken not to touch the cornea, which could cause further eye injury. Careful aseptic technique is needed to prevent infection.

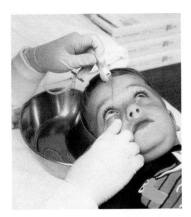

Figure 7-7 *Eye irrigation.*

SKILL 7-6 Performing an Eye Irrigation

PREPARATION

1. Check the physician's orders for the type of fluid and the volume to be used (most often sterile normal saline).
2. The child will need to be held in position for this procedure. An assistant can hold the child supine with the body over the child's, keeping the child's head turned slightly so that the eye to be irrigated is lower than the other eye.
   RATIONALE: *This method is used to avoid cross-contamination of the eye not being irrigated.*
3. Attach the IV tubing to the bag of room temperature normal saline. Purge the line, but keep the tip covered.

EQUIPMENT AND SUPPLIES

- Absorbent pads
- Irrigation solution and tubing
- Basin

PROCEDURE: *Sterile Gloves*

1. Place absorbent pads under the child's head, neck, and shoulders, using towels for extra absorption. Place an emesis basin under the lower eye to catch drainage.
2. Don gloves.
3. Using the thumb and forefinger of the dominant hand, gently separate the child's lids.
4. Remove the cover from the IV tubing. Open the clamp midway, pointing the stream of fluid into the lower conjunctival sac from the inner to the outer canthus. Periodically turn off the stream of solution and have the child close the eye.
   RATIONALE: *This procedure allows the solution to also move into the upper conjunctival area.*
5. When the irrigation has been completed, dry the child's eye gently with gauze or a cotton ball from the inner to the outer canthus.
6. Assess the return for color, odor, and character.

Otic Medication

Otic medications, which are available in liquid form, are placed in the external ear canal using a dropper. Otic drops are sometimes applied to soften cerumen, enabling it to be cleansed from the canal. The ear canal is not treated with sterile technique unless the tympanic membrane is ruptured and draining.

SKILL 7-7 Administering an Otic Medication

PREPARATION

1. Gather supplies.

EQUIPMENT AND SUPPLIES

- Medication
- Cotton ball

PROCEDURE: *Clean Gloves*

1. Have another nurse, an assistant, or the parent restrain the child in a supine position with the head turned as appropriate for administration (Figure 7-8).

2. Don gloves.

3. *For the child less than 3 years of age:* Gently pull the pinna straight back and downward to straighten the ear canal.
   For the older child: Pull the pinna back and upward.

4. When the pinna is in the proper position, instill the drops into the ear.

5. Keep the child in the same position for a few minutes. Gently rub the area just anterior to the ear to facilitate drainage of the medication into the ear canal. If desired, a cotton ball may be loosely placed in the ear to promote retention of the medication.

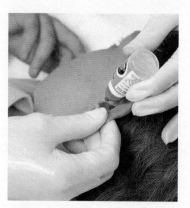

Figure 7-8 *Administering an otic medication.*

Ear Irrigation

Irrigation of the ear is performed to remove cerumen or a foreign body. Frequently the child has symptoms of otitis media but the canal cannot be visualized. Always ask the parent if there has been any drainage from the ear and examine the ear with an otoscope (see Chapter 4 of *Pediatric Nursing: Caring for Children, Third Edition,* for a description of proper use of the otoscope and normal ear landmarks). If there is drainage, contact the physician before irrigating the ear. Be sure to check with the otoscope after about 1 minute of irrigation to observe the effects of treatment.

SKILL 7-8 Performing an Ear Irrigation

PREPARATION

1. Check the physician's orders for the type of fluid to be administered.

EQUIPMENT AND SUPPLIES

- Ordered solution, warmed to room temperature
- Irrigating syringe (bulb or Asepto) with tubing or water pik
- Clean gloves
- Absorbent pads
- Basin

PROCEDURE: *Clean Gloves*

1. Examine the ear with an otoscope.
   RATIONALE: *The tympanic membrane should be intact before the irrigation is performed.*

2. Position the child on the back. Don gloves. For the child less than 3 years of age, gently pull the pinna straight back and slightly downward. For the older child, pull the pinna back and upward.
   RATIONALE: *These maneuvers straighten the ear canal.*

3. Place an emesis basin under the ear to be irrigated. Place a waterproof pad on the bed under the head (Figure 7-9).

4. Draw 20 mL of warm ordered solution into a syringe with the tubing attached.

5. Gently flush the solution into the ear canal, catching the draining fluid with the emesis basin.

6. Alternately, use a water pik at the lowest setting to flush the ear.

7. Repeat according to prescriber's orders.

8. Reexamine the ear with an otoscope and record changes from the treatment.

9. Dry the child's ear, cheek, and neck.

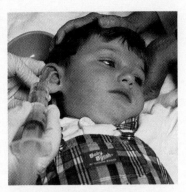

Figure 7-9 *Ear irrigation.*

Nasal Medication

Medications instilled into the nares drain into the back of the mouth and throat, and may cause sensations of difficulty in breathing, tickling, or bad taste. After instillation of the drops, the child should be observed for choking or vomiting. Saline nose drops are sometimes given to young infants who have respiratory disorders to clear the nasal passages.

SKILL 7-9 Administering a Nasal Medication

EQUIPMENT AND SUPPLIES

- Medication

PROCEDURE: *Clean Gloves*

1. Place the child in a supine position with the head hyperextended over the parent's lap or over the edge of the examination table or bed.

2. Don gloves.

3. Instill the drops into the nostrils.

4. Keep the child in the same position for at least 5 minutes to allow the medication to contact the nasal mucosa.

Aerosol Therapy

Aerosol therapy is used when medication must be deposited directly into the airway. Bronchodilators, steroids, and antibiotics can be administered to children in aerosol form. Several methods are used to provide aerosol therapy, including mist tents with medications added to a reservoir, intermittent positive pressure breathing machines, or nebulizers. The most common aerosol therapy for children is the metered dose inhaler (MDI) commonly used in treatment of asthma (see Chapter 13 of *Pediatric Nursing: Caring for Children, Third Edition*, for a description of this treatment for asthma). Because nebulizers are the type of aerosol treatment commonly used in the hospital and administered by nurses, their use is also described here.

SKILL 7-10 Administering Nebulizer Aerosol Therapy

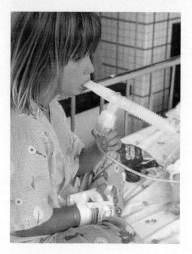

Figure 7-10 *This child has been taught to use a nebulizer for treatment of her asthma in the hospital. After explanation and demonstration by the nurse, she now independently and effectively completes the treatment.*

PREPARATION

1. The dose of the medication is based on the child's weight. The medication is placed in the cup of the aerosol kit; 2 to 3 mL of normal saline can be added as a diluent if ordered.

2. Perform a baseline assessment, including heart and respiratory rates, breath sounds, and respiratory effort.

EQUIPMENT AND SUPPLIES

- Reservoir
- Mouthpiece or blow-by tubing (depending on child's age)
- Portable nebulizing machine or tubing to hook to oxygen supply

PROCEDURE

1. Place the mask on the child.

2. Give an assistant or the parent the tubing for blow-by, or have the child put the mouthpiece in the mouth (Figure 7-10).

3. Attach the oxygen tubing to the oxygen flowmeter at 6–7 L/min.

4. Have the child take deep breaths during the treatment.

5. The aerosol administration should last about 10 minutes. Reassess the child's condition after the therapy.

HOME CARE CONSIDERATIONS

When a child is using a metered dose inhaler, observe the child's self-administration technique on occasional home and office visits. Offer teaching to improve the use and effectiveness of the inhaler, if needed. Record your observations and teaching and follow up on a later visit.

Metered Dose Inhaler

Metered dose inhalers (MDIs) are small canister devices with a mouthpiece used to treat asthma in the home setting. They may be used on a regular basis or during times of respiratory distress.

SKILL 7-11 Using a Metered Dose Inhaler

EQUIPMENT AND SUPPLIES

- Inhaler with medication

PROCEDURE

1. Insert the canister into the mouthpiece.

2. Have the child take a deep breath of room air, inhaling and exhaling completely.

3. Ask the child to close the lips tightly over the MDI mouthpiece, and then inhale deeply and slowly through the mouth.

4. Depress the canister one time while the child is inhaling; one dose of medication will be inhaled.

5. Have the child hold his or her breath for about 5 to 10 seconds to enable medication to reach the lungs.

6. MDIs may have reservoirs, spacers, or extenders for those children having difficulty holding their breath long enough or closing their mouths securely over the mouthpiece.

Topical Therapy

Children with deep partial thickness burns have regular dressing changes and debridement during the healing process. A topical antibiotic cream such as silvadene is used as a barrier to infectious organisms.

PREPARATION

1. Explain the procedure to the child and parent and why it is needed. Encourage the parent to provide a distracting activity, such as reading a story or watching a video, during the dressing change.

2. Check the physician's orders. Because burn care is a painful procedure, check for pain medication orders and administer medication at least 30 to 60 minutes before starting burn care. Conscious sedation may be used for some debridement procedures.
   RATIONALE: *Medication must be administered so that peak action occurs during the burn dressing change.*

3. Wash hands. An assistant may need to hold the child and the burned extremity during care.

EQUIPMENT AND SUPPLIES

- Basin
- Sterile normal saline solution
- Large supply of 4 × 4 gauze pads
- Forceps
- Scissors
- Sterile tongue blade
- Prescribed topical medication
- Tape
- Absorbent pad

PROCEDURE: *Clean and Sterile Gloves*

1. Place the absorbent pad under the area to be cleaned. Put on clean gloves. Soak the wound for about 10 minutes in normal saline solution, or apply a wet dressing to the area. Remove the gloves
   RATIONALE: *This method will soften the wound and make it easier to remove the old dressing.*

2. Using sterile gloves, wash the burn with the gauze pads and sterile normal saline to remove any medication and crusting. Use a firm, circular motion, moving from the inside to the outer edges. Bleeding may occur, but this is a sign of healing, healthy tissue. Rinse with normal saline solution. Pat dry with sterile gauze.
   RATIONALE: *The injured skin secretes serous fluid that forms a tough leathery layer called eschar. This layer must be removed to promote healing.*

3. Some children are placed in a whirlpool bath to soften the eschar and increase circulation.

4. Remove (per physician's orders) any loose or dead skin around the burn's edges by gently lifting it with the forceps and snipping it. This is not painful to the child. Rinse and dry again.
   RATIONALE: *Debridement speeds the healing process.*

5. Place a thin layer of prescribed medication (about 1/8-in. thick) on the burn or gauze with fingers or a sterile tongue blade.

6. Place the medicated gauze on the burn and cover with a dry, sterile dressing.

Rectal Medication

Rectal administration is sometimes used when the oral route is contraindicated. Although absorption is less reliable than with oral preparations, many medications, such as acetaminophen, aspirin, antiemetics, analgesics, and sedatives, come in suppository form.

SKILL 7-13 Administering a Rectal Medication

PREPARATION

1. If the suppository is to be halved, cut it lengthwise.

EQUIPMENT AND SUPPLIES

- Water-soluble lubricant
- Suppository

PROCEDURE: *Clean Gloves*

1. Have another nurse, an assistant, or the parent hold the child in a side-lying or (if small enough) a prone position on the parent's lap.

2. Don gloves.

3. Slightly lubricate the tapered tip of the suppository. Using either the index finder (in children over 3 years of age) or the little finger (in infants and toddlers), gently insert the suppository into the child's rectum, just beyond the internal sphincter.
   RATIONALE: *Lubrication provides for easy insertion and minimal trauma to the mucous membranes. The child's rectum is small in size. Insertion past the sphincter allows the medication to stay in place for absorption.*

4. Hold the buttocks together for 5 to 10 minutes, until the urge to expel the medication has passed.

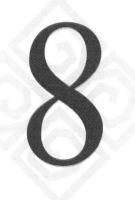

8

Intravenous Access

Chapter Outline

Peripheral Vascular Access

In both infants and children, veins of the extremities are used for venous access. Scalp veins may also be used in infants.

Over-the-needle catheters (19 to 27 gauge) are preferred for infants and children. The size of the catheter is determined by the size of both the child and the vein. For example, a 24-gauge catheter is used for a newborn; a 20- to 22-gauge catheter is used for an older infant, toddler, or school-age child. A butterfly needle (23 gauge) may be used in certain situations, such as when accessing a scalp vein in an infant or during an emergency for peripheral access in a young child. Use of a butterfly needle should be considered a temporary measure, with continued effort made to achieve more stable and secure venous access.

Choice of Site

Scalp

Scalp veins are used when other access cannot be obtained (Figure 8-1). Protect the site by covering it with a plastic medication cup secured with tape.

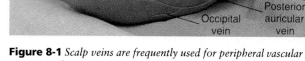

Figure 8-1 *Scalp veins are frequently used for peripheral vascular access in infants.*

Extremities

Veins of the antecubital fossa or forearm are usually the best sites for venous access because they are highly visible; however, the dorsum of the hand and foot also may be used.

Special Considerations

- Avoid using the foot veins as a site in children who are walking.

- Avoid using the child's dominant hand or the hand used by an infant for finger sucking or blanket holding.

- If two sites are needed, do not use both antecubital veins, because the child will be rendered helpless.

- Use padded armboards as splints to decrease mobility of the extremity.

- Use gauze under tape or tape over tape to decrease skin contact with adhesive tape.

SKILL 8-1 Accessing a Peripheral Vein

PREPARATION: *Clean Gloves*

1. Don gloves.

2. Place and maintain the child in a supine position with the help of an assistant. Have the assistant lean over the child to control the child's body and extend the extremity to be used. An alternative to human restraint is to use a papoose board (see Chapter 2).

3. If a scalp vein is to be used, place a rubber band around the infant's head to serve as a tourniquet to distend the veins. If the extremities are to be used, place the tourniquet proximal to the desired vein to distend it. If necessary, hold the extremity below heart level, gently rub or tap the vein, or apply a warm compress to promote dilation of the vein.

4. Locate the vein by inspection (wiping with alcohol will make the vein shine) or palpation.

5. If you are using an extremity, apply an armboard or footboard. Relocate the vein.

6. *If using the antecubital fossa:* Slightly hyperextend the child's elbow and pronate the arm. Secure the arm to the armboard by applying tape above the elbow and at the wrist.

7. *If using the dorsum of the hand:* Place the child's hand on the armboard, palmar side down, with the fingers wrapped around the distal edge (Figure 8-2). Apply tape over the fingers, then around the thumb separately. Next apply tape at the wrist. A gauze roll may be placed under the wrist to increase flexion.

   RATIONALE: *Positioning to avoid injury is an important nursing role.*

8. *If using the foot:* Apply the footboard to the child's foot, which is dorsiflexed. Apply tape across the toes, instep, and ankle. Use gauze as needed under the lateral malleolus.

EQUIPMENT AND SUPPLIES

- Tourniquet
- Alcohol or povidone-iodine
- Different-size armboards
- IV catheter (depends on size of vein)
- T connector that has been flushed and attached to normal saline–filled syringe
- IV tubing and bag with solution

PROCEDURE: *Clean Gloves*

1. Apply gloves.

2. Clean the skin with alcohol or povidone-iodine using an outward circular motion. Let each area dry before continuing. Apply the tourniquet. Hold the skin taut, gently pulling with your thumb just distal to the site of the puncture.

3. Puncture the skin with the catheter, with the bevel side up, positioned at a 15-degree angle and aimed at the vein in the direction of the blood flow. When blood appears, gently slide the catheter into the vein. Release the tourniquet. Remove the stylette.

4. Attach the normal saline–filled T connector and attempt to flush the catheter. If it flushes easily, tape the catheter in place, using a V pattern around the catheter itself. Further secure the catheter with gauze and tape (taking care not to cover the area proximal to the site completely). Alternately, a transparent dressing can be used over the site.

   RATIONALE: *Wrapping techniques promote intactness of the line and allow for visualization of the site for signs of infiltration or phlebitis.*

5. Write the date, time, catheter size, and initials on a piece of tape and place it on the dressing.

   RATIONALE: *Agencies set policies about how long an IV line can be kept in place. Accurate documentation and labeling ensure changes on schedule to avoid infections.*

6. The T connector can be hooked up to a heparin lock or used immediately for fluid or medication infusion.

(See Chapter 6 for further explanation of intravenous access to obtain a blood sample.)

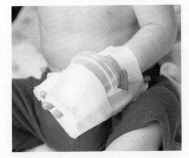

Figure 8-2 *This intravenous site on a hand has been placed on an armboard, securely wrapped, and covered with part of a plastic cup to prevent the child from disrupting the line.*

Medication Lock

The medication lock is a small device placed on the IV catheter and taped to secure. It maintains the IV site for future use when not hooked to a running IV infusion. Some agencies use normal saline, whereas others use heparin solution to maintain patency of medication locks (this is more commonly done with older children than with infants). Know and follow agency policy.

SKILL 8-2 Attaching a Medication Lock Cap to an IV Infusion

PREPARATION

1. Verify order.

2. Record intake of intravenous fluid for documentation

RESEARCH CONSIDERATIONS

Several nursing studies have been performed to measure the effectiveness of heparin versus saline flushes for intravenous lines in children. Different findings and conclusions have failed to give clear guidance to nurses and agencies about the best method. Therefore, agencies may set different policies about this procedure. Evidence suggests that small-gauge IV lines (such as 24-gauge lines) may be maintained more successfully with heparin; larger lines may be maintained with either saline or heparin. Check on policy in your clinical agency.

EQUIPMENT AND SUPPLIES

- Syringe filled with 1 mL of prepackaged heparin flush solution (10 U/mL)
- Syringe with 2 mL of sterile normal saline
- Luer-lok male adapter

PROCEDURE: *Clean Gloves*

1. Prime the adaptor (fill it, being sure to prevent air pockets) with the heparin flush solution. Maintain sterility of the adaptor tip that will be inserted into the intravenous line.

2. Save the rest of the heparin flush solution to use when the lok is inserted into the IV tubing.

3. Don gloves.

4. Be sure the IV line is securely taped in place (Figure 8-3A). Check the patency of the IV tubing by flushing with 2 mL of sterile normal saline. Be sure there is no redness, swelling, pallor, coolness, or pain at the IV site.

5. Clamp the T connector on the IV line to prevent outflow of blood.

6. Remove the IV tubing from the line and quickly place a primed catheter cap on the T connector.

7. Open the clamp. Insert the heparin flush solution or saline and slowly flush the adaptor.

8. Remove the syringe and clamp the medication lock.

9. Secure the medication lock with tape and cover with an elastic bandage (Figure 8-3B).

10. Flush the line every 8 hours with heparin flush solution or as determined by agency policy.

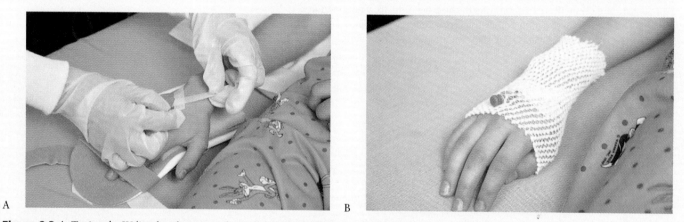

A   B

Figure 8-3 *A, Taping the IV line for placement of a medication lock. B, Medication lock in place.*

SKILL 8-3 Infusing Medication: Medication Lock in Place

PREPARATION

1. Verify order.

2. Calculate and check medication dosage.

EQUIPMENT AND SUPPLIES

- Alcohol swabs
- 19- to 27-gauge needle or needleless system
- Two syringes filled with 2 mL of normal saline with 19- to 27-gauge needles or needless system
- Medication ordered
- Syringe with 1 mL of heparin flush solution (10 U/mL) or sterile normal saline

PROCEDURE: *Clean Gloves*

1. Don gloves

2. Prepare the medication to be administered.

3. Clean the catheter cap with alcohol. Unclamp the medication lock.

4. Check the patency of the IV tubing by flushing it with normal saline. Check the catheter tip site for swelling.

5. If the IV line is patent and operating, apply the new syringe or needless system on the distal end of the IV tubing through the cap after cleaning its surface.

    RATIONALE: *Recessed needles or needleless systems are recommended when available to promote safety.*

6. Secure the IV tubing and connection area in place with tape.

7. Administer the infusion of medication according to the prescriber's orders.

8. Be sure to follow the infusion with 10 to 20 mL of IV fluid so no medication remains in the tubing.

9. After completion of the infusion, discard used equipment into a puncture-proof container according to standard precaution recommendations.

10. If the IV tubing is to be used again, cover it with a clean needle system to ensure sterility.

11. Clean the catheter cap with alcohol.

12. Flush first with 2 mL of normal saline and follow with the heparin flush solution if heparin is to be used (as in the preceding procedure). Clamp the medication lock and secure it in place.

SKILL 8-4 Administering an IV Push Bolus of Medication: Medication Lock in Place

PREPARATION

1. Check order.

2. Calculate and check medication dosage.

EQUIPMENT AND SUPPLIES

- Alcohol swabs
- Two 1- to 2-mL syringes filled with normal saline with 19- to 25-gauge needles or needleless system
- Syringe filled with 1 mL of heparin flush solution (10 U/mL) or sterile normal saline
- Medication in syringe covered with 19- to 25-gauge needle

PROCEDURE: *Clean Gloves*

1. Don gloves.

2. Clean the catheter cap with alcohol. Unclamp the medication lock.

3. Pierce the catheter cap with a normal saline–filled syringe.

4. Flush the line with 2 mL of normal saline to check patency.

5. Remove the syringe and needle.

6. Insert the medication syringe through the catheter cap and administer according to the prescriber's orders. Check a medication resource book or call the hospital pharmacy to determine the rate of administration. When all medication has been administered, remove the syringe.

7. Flush the line with the 2 mL of normal saline, followed by the heparin flush solution if the latter is used. Clamp and secure the medication line.

8. Discard the equipment in a puncture-proof container according to standard precaution recommendations.

Intravenous Infusion

The amount of fluid to be administered to a child is based on the child's weight and pathophysiologic state. It is recommended that fluids be given to the infant or child through an infusion pump (Figure 8-4), as this device allows for a more accurate setting of flow rates than does gravity. Maintenance fluid requirements are based on the child's weight (see Table 8-1).

Pumps

An infusion pump can be used to control the administration of small volumes of fluid, blood, medication, and total parenteral nutrition. A smaller syringe pump (Figure 8-5) can be attached directly to the lowest port on the IV tubing for immediate infusion of medication.

It is important to be familiar with the type of infusion pump used at your institution. Be sure to set controls for both the amount of fluid to be infused and the rate of infusion. Check the pump frequently to be certain it is programmed and working correctly.

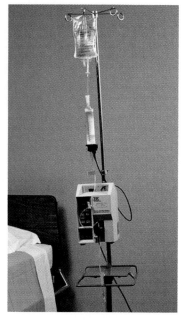

Figure 8-4 *IV setup with infusion pump.*

Figure 8-5 *Syringe pump.*

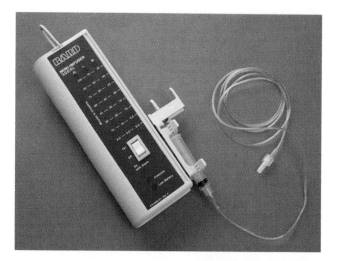

TABLE 8-1	Pediatric Maintenance Fluid Requirements
Weight (kg)	**Fluid Requirements**
0–10	100 mL/kg/24 hr
10–20	1000 mL + 50 mL/kg/24 hr for each kg between 11 and 20
20–70	1500 mL + 20 mL/kg/24 hr for each kg between 21 and 70
Over 70	2500 mL/24 hr (adult requirement)

SKILL 8-5 Administering IV Fluids

PREPARATION

1. Check the fluid order for type of fluid and infusion rate. Compare with the fluid needs of the child (see Chapter 10 in *Pediatric Nursing: Caring for Children, Third Edition,* for calculating children's maintenance and replacement fluids).

2. Gather supplies.

EQUIPMENT AND SUPPLIES

- Intravenous fluid
- Tubing
- Infusion pump
- Tape and labels

PROCEDURE: *Clean Gloves*

1. Check the bag or bottle for leaks, expiration date, impurities, or color changes.
2. Open tubing package. Make sure that the tubing is clamped off.
3. Remove the protective covering from the insertion piece (spike). Place the insertion piece into the entry port of the bag or bottle. Invert the bag or bottle and hang it on a pole.
4. Pinch the drip chamber (it should be no more than one-half full). Direct the distal end of the tubing into a clean receptacle, maintaining sterility of the end. Open the clamp and let the fluid run through the length of the tubing. Tap the tubing at each port to remove any trapped air.
5. Close the clamp, recap the sterile end, and check the entire length of tubing for air bubbles. The tubing is now primed and ready for use.
6. If a volume control chamber (Soluset or Metriset) is used, first attach it to the bag or bottle. Close the clamp that is closest to the fluid and the one that is distal to the chamber. Open the top clamp.
7. Let about 50 mL into the chamber and then close the clamp. Pinch the drip chamber as above. Open the distal clamp, and continue to purge the tubing (as described above).
8. If using a pump, check the manufacturer's guidelines for purging the tubing.
9. Mark the bottle or bag with label and tape that lists child's identifying information, type of infusion, flow rate, and date and time of preparation.
10. Bring the primed intravenous infusion to the child.
11. Don gloves.
12. If replacing a bag that is finished, clamp tubing on the venous line and on the existing tubing before removing the old tubing.
13. Check the IV site carefully for leakage, redness, pallor, swelling, and pain.
14. Remove the cover on the end of the IV tubing, maintaining sterility of the tip.
15. Place the tip into the existing IV line.
16. Unclamp the IV line and the tubing and begin the flow of fluid.
17. Check the site carefully for leakage, redness, pallor, swelling, and pain as the infusion begins. Repeat assessments according to agency policy.
18. Document the application of a new bag and update the intake record of the child by including fluid from the bag that has been infused.

Guidelines for Infusion of IV Fluids

Rules for determining flow rate for instilling IV fluids via gravity are based on the drip factor of the IV tubing being used.

Microdrip Tubing

Manufacturer	Drops/mL
All major manufacturers	60 drops (gtt) = 1 mL

FORMULA
mL/hr = gtt/min

EXAMPLE
1,000 mL/8 hr = 125 mL/hr = 125 gtt/min

Macrodrip Tubing

Manufacturer	Drops/mL
Abbot	15 gtt = 1 mL
Baxter	10 gtt = 1 mL

FORMULA

Total volume × Drop factor/Infusion time in minutes = Drops/minute

EXAMPLE

1,000 mL × 10 (Travenol)/8 hr (480 min) = 21 gtt/min

Blood Administration

To safely administer blood or blood products to the infant or child, be aware of the protocols followed at your institution. Ensure that an informed consent for administration is present in the chart. Because hypersensitivity reactions can occur and other side effects can be severe, administration of blood is approached with many nursing cautions. Be sure to take vital signs and monitor the child closely. Follow instructions from the blood bank and other resources for correct administration of blood products, such as frozen plasma, cryoprecipitate, and clotting factors.

NURSING ALERT

Blood is administered according to the physician's orders. However, a bag should never remain hanging longer than 4 hours. Do not use the blood line for any other infusions. If a medication must be administered by that line, turn off the infusion, flush the line with normal saline, administer the medication, flush the line again with normal saline, and then restart the blood infusion.

SKILL 8-6 Administering Blood or Blood Products

PREPARATION

1. Identify the bag to be used and compare it with the requisition (type, Rh factor, patient number, blood donor number) and the child's identification bracelet. Do this step with another nurse at the bedside. Both nurses are responsible for signing the slips as the transfusers.
   RATIONALE: *Administration of blood has serious implications for damage to the patient. Having two nurses check minimizes the opportunity for error.*

2. Check the blood for any bubbles, dark areas, or sediment.
   RATIONALE: *These discolorations can indicate that the blood is old or has not been properly maintained.*

3. Ask the child or family about previous transfusions, especially any history of allergic reactions.

4. Take the child's vital signs, including pulse, respiratory rate, temperature, and blood pressure.
   RATIONALE: *Baseline vital signs may be useful for comparison later in the procedure.*

5. When estimating preparation time, keep in mind that blood must be hung within 20 to 30 minutes after being removed from the blood bank refrigerator. For trauma patients who need massive transfusions, the bag should be warmed to 37°C (99°F) (only an approved blood warmer should be used).

6. Use the correct tubing for the blood product being administered. A Y blood administration set is preferred. If a Y setup is used, hang normal saline at the extra connector.

EQUIPMENT AND SUPPLIES

- Blood product
- Y tubing and bag of normal saline
- Normal saline flush solution
- Sterile needle or needleless system
- Intravenous line in place with 18-gauge needle or larger

PROCEDURE: *Clean or Sterile Gloves*

1. Take the child's baseline vital signs.

2. Verify the type and cross-match data on the blood with another registered nurse.

3. Attach the blood bag to one end of the Y tubing. Flush the line with normal saline attached to the other side of the Y tubing.

   RATIONALE: *Checking the line for patency and using normal saline to prevent incompatibilities contributes to safe infusion.*

4. Clamp off the tubing, keeping the distal end covered.

5. Disconnect it, covering the hub with a sterile needle or needleless system to keep it sterile. Flush the child's IV line with normal saline to ensure its patency.

6. Attach the blood tubing.

7. Slowly open the clamp on tubing, adjusting the flow with the roller. Start the transfusion slowly.

8. The flow rate may be increased if no reaction is noted.

   RATIONALE: *Most reactions occur within 20 minutes.*

9. Closely monitor the child's vital signs and response. Vital signs should be taken every 5 minutes for the first 15 minutes, every 15 minutes during the first hour, then hourly until the transfusion is complete (*or* follow your hospital's protocol).

10. If the child develops any sign of a transfusion reaction (Table 8-2), stop the transfusion, change the IV to normal saline, and notify the physician immediately.

11. After the administration of blood, flush the line with normal saline and connect the IV fluid ordered by the physician. Place the used blood bag and tubing in a plastic bag, seal it, and return it to the blood bank with copies of the transfusion information sheet.

    RATIONALE: *This is a method of verification of the blood use and the patient data.*

12. Document all vital signs, responses, and interventions.

HOME CARE CONSIDERATIONS

When a child receives a transfusion of blood or blood products, administration of immunizations must be delayed for several months afterward. Measles and varicella vaccines are particularly ineffective following blood transfusions. Be sure to let parents know and provide in writing the type of product used (whole blood, packed red cell, frozen plasma, etc), and the date of the infusion. Instruct them to take this information with them when they next visit their regular care provider so that adaptations in immunization administration may be implemented if needed.

TABLE 8-2	Transfusion Reactions	
Type of Reaction	**Cause**	**Description**
Allergic	Caused by immune response to protein in blood	Signs and symptoms may include rash, itching, urticaria, wheezing, laryngospasm, edema, and/or anaphylaxis
Febrile or septic	Usually a result of contamination of blood; may also be caused by idiopathic conditions	Signs and symptoms include chills, fever, headache, decreased blood pressure, nausea and/or vomiting, and leg or back pain
Hemolytic	Caused by incompatibility of child's blood with donor blood, history of multiple transfusions, or infusion with a solution containing dextrose or other additives	Signs and symptoms include anxiety or restlessness, fever, chills, chest pain, cyanosis, change in vital signs with increased heart and respiratory rates or with decreased blood pressure and/or hematuria; can progress to shock and anuria if not treated promptly
Circulatory overload	Results from infusion of excessive amounts of fluid or too rapid administration	Signs and symptoms include labored breathing, chest or lower back pain, productive cough with rales heard on auscultation, and distended neck veins; central venous pressure may increase

SKILL 8-7 Total Parenteral Nutrition

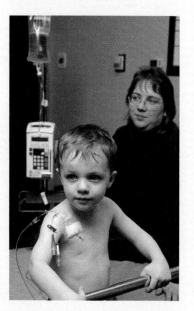

Figure 8-6 *This child is receiving TPN.*

Total parenteral nutrition (TPN) is the administration of a nutritionally complete formula into a large central vein (see Figure 8-6). TPN is used for children who cannot tolerate gastrointestinal feeding. Children with disorders such as chronic intestinal obstruction, short bowel syndrome, chronic diarrhea, or tumors may require TPN. (The care of these disorders is discussed in Chapters 16 and 17 of *Pediatric Nursing: Caring for Children, Third Edition*.)

Hyperalimentation solutions (TPN and lipid emulsions) are delivered by separate pumps and connector tubes. The child who is receiving TPN has a central venous catheter in place. Solutions and tubes must be changed every 24 hours using strict aseptic technique. Tips and connecting points must be sterile. A filter is used for infusion. Nursing responsibilities when caring for a child receiving TPN are outlined in Table 8-3.

TABLE 8-3	Caring for the Child Receiving TPN

- Monitor intake and output. Changes may indicate fluid and electrolyte disturbances.
- Weigh the child daily.
- Assess the IV site. Watch for signs of redness, irritation, or infection. Change the dressing according to hospital protocol (see the procedure for managing a central venous catheter site in this unit).
- Use the infusion site only for TPN solutions or keep the line open with normal saline. Do not use the line for medications or other infusions.
- Make sure to set each pump correctly, noting the volume and rate of each infusion.
- Check laboratory values, especially glucose, minerals, electrolytes, liver function (bilirubin, alkaline phosphatase), proteins, and triglycerides.
- Note any change in glucose levels:
  1. During the first few days, the high concentration of glucose administration may lead to hyperglycemia. Inform the physician of high blood glucose levels. Insulin may be needed to help the body adjust to the formula.
  2. If hyperalimentation is discontinued abruptly, the child may become hypoglycemic. Be aware of the signs and symptoms of hypoglycemia (see Chapter 22 of Ball and Bindler's *Pediatric Nursing*). Notify the physician if the child's blood glucose level is low.

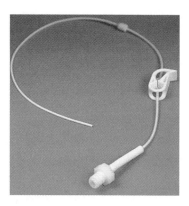

Figure 8-7 *Broviac catheter.*

Central Venous Catheters

A central venous catheter is surgically placed when long-term access is needed, such as for total parenteral nutrition, administration of antibiotics, or chemotherapy. Usually the subclavian vein is accessed and the catheter is threaded into the right atrium.

The most common catheter used for children is the Broviac catheter (Figure 8-7), which can have a single, double, or triple lumen. Other catheters such as the Hickman may be used with older children. Peripherally inserted central catheter (PICC) lines are also common in children. Catheter lines require flushing; Broviac catheters are flushed once a day, both at home and in the hospital, if they are not accessed for infusions. For flushing, 5 mL of heparin flush solution is used. Consult agency policies for frequency of flushing in particular institutions. In addition, the site requires care, as described in the following procedure.

Site Management

The catheter site is covered with a clear occlusive dressing that should be changed under sterile conditions two to three times a week according to agency protocol.

SKILL 8-8 Managing a Central Venous Catheter Site

PREPARATION

1. Gather necessary supplies.
2. Evaluate the dressing and visible skin at the catheter site.

EQUIPMENT AND SUPPLIES

- Peroxide-saturated cotton swabs
- Alcohol swabs
- Providone-iodine swabs
- Central venous catheter kit
- Sterile occlusive dressing

PROCEDURE: *Clean and Sterile Gloves (if not using a kit with gloves enclosed)*

1. Open the kit. Don mask and clean gloves.
2. Remove the current dressing, working from the edges toward the center. Discard the old dressing and gloves.
3. Wash hands and don the sterile gloves. Clean site with sterile half-strength peroxide-saturated cotton swabs in an outward circular motion from the point of entry, using one swab for each motion and then changing to a clean one. Clean the area again with alcohol swabs three times, then povidone-iodine swabs, using the same technique.
4. Clean the catheter tubing from the exit site to the cap.
5. Let dry. Apply antibacterial ointment around the exit site. Place a small sterile gauze over and under the catheter insertion site. Cover with a sterile occlusive dressing.
6. Write the date, time, and initials on a piece of tape and place it on the dressing.

SKILL 8-9 Accessing a Central Venous Catheter

A central line may be accessed for the drawing of blood samples. The following describes the single-syringe method.

PREPARATION

1. Check the physician's order for the blood tests to be done.

   RATIONALE: *It is recommended that the catheter be accessed no more than twice a day to minimize chance of infection.*

2. Locate an assistant to open and close the clamps as necessary and put the blood in tubes while you are flushing the line.

EQUIPMENT AND SUPPLIES

- Sterile 4 × 4 gauze pad
- Povidone-iodine solution
- Cotton-tipped swabs

- Appropriate blood collection tubes
- 19- to 27-gauge needles for transferring blood to tubes
- Padded clamp (if a clamp is not attached to tubing)

For each port accessed:

- Syringe filled with 5 to 6 mL of normal saline
- Syringe filled with 20 mL normal saline
- Syringe filled with 2 to 3 mL of heparin flush solution (10 U/mL)
- 5- to 6-mL empty syringe (to draw and discard initial blood)
- Syringes for blood samples
- Luer-lok or Broviac catheter cap

PROCEDURE: *Sterile Gloves*

1. Unpin the catheter from the child's clothes. Remove any tape. Open a sterile 4 × 4 gauze pad to serve as a clean work area. Don sterile gloves. Place the gauze under the catheter connection. If the intravenous solution is infusing, turn it off (Figure 8-8).

2. Clean the connection site with povidine-iodine. Use three swabs, and clean for a total of 2 minutes. Let the connection site dry for an additional 20 seconds.

3. Make sure the catheter is clamped. Remove the catheter cap or infusion tubing, maintaining sterility. Flush the catheter with 2 to 5 mL of normal saline to ensure patency. Slowly aspirate 3 to 5 mL of blood. Clamp the catheter and discard the syringe. Using another 10-mL syringe, aspirate the amount of blood necessary. Remove the blood-filled syringe and cover with a 19-gauge needle or needleless system. Have the assistant use that syringe to fill the blood collection tubes. Meanwhile, attach the syringe filled with normal saline. Flush the line first with the 20 mL of normal saline, then with the prepared heparin flush solution.

4. Clamp the catheter and remove the flush syringe. Connect the infusion solution or cover the port with a sterile protector.

5. Secure the catheter to the child's clothing. Remove the gloves and wash hands.

6. Ensure that blood specimens are labeled properly, kept at proper temperature, and transported to the laboratory.

Figure 8-8 *The nurse uses sterile technique and carefully examines the central line to plan access from the proper port.*

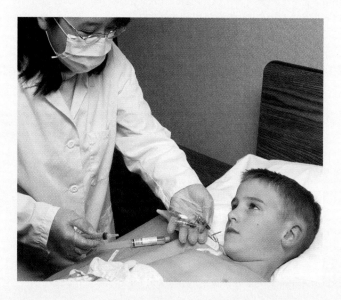

SKILL 8-10 Implanted Ports

Implanted ports are used most often for children and adolescents who require long-term venous access. The stainless steel port has a self-sealing rubber septum and is surgically implanted under the skin over a bony prominence, most often the clavicle. The catheter is then inserted into the vein that leads to the right atrium. Entry is gained by piercing the skin directly over the port with a specially designed needle (Figure 8-9). Sterile gloves, mask, and gown are worn when accessing the site.

The Port-a-Cath is used commonly in pediatrics.

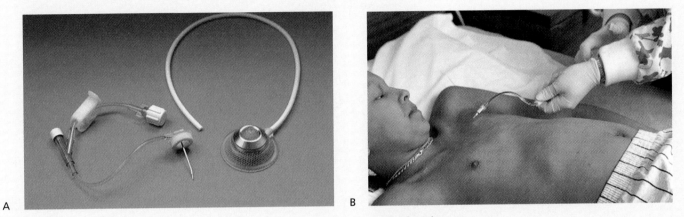

A   B

Figure 8-9 *A, Huber needle. B, Nurse drawing blood from an adolescent who has an implanted port.*

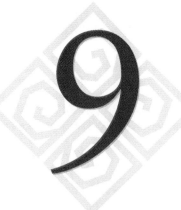

Pain Assessment and Management

Chapter Outline

Pain Assessment

Pain is considered the fifth vital sign, and every child has the right to be assessed for pain and receive pain management. The goal of pain assessment is to provide accurate information about the location and intensity of pain and its effects on the child's functioning. Various pain scales have been developed to assess pain in children. Some pain assessment scales rely on the nurse's observation of the child's behavior if the child is nonverbal. Most scales depend on the child's report of pain intensity. For more information, refer to Chapter 9 in *Pediatric Nursing: Caring for Children, Third Edition*.

SKILL 9-1 Selected Pediatric Pain Scales

NEONATAL INFANT PAIN SCALE (NIPS)

- Use in preterm and term infants up to 6 weeks after birth.
- Observe the infant's facial expression, cry quality, breathing pattern, arm and leg position, and state of arousal (Table 9-1).

TABLE 9-1	Neonatal Infant Pain Scale (NIPS)
Characteristic	**Scoring Criteria**
Facial Expression 0 = Relaxed muscles 1 = Grimace	■ Restful face with neutral expression ■ Tight facial muscles; furrowed brow, chin, and jaw (Note: At low gestational ages, infants may have no facial expression.)
Cry 0 = No cry 1 = Whimper 2 = Vigorous cry	■ Quiet, not crying ■ Mild moaning, intermittent cry ■ Loud screaming, rising, shrill, and continuous (Note: Silent cry may be scored if infant is intubated, as indicated by obvious facial movements.)
Breathing Patterns 0 = Relaxed 1 = Change in breathing	■ Relaxed, usual breathing pattern maintained ■ Change in breathing, irregular, faster than usual, gagging, or holding breath
Arm Movements 0 = Relaxed/restrained 1 = Flexed/extended	■ Relaxed, no muscle rigidity, occasional random (with soft restraints) movements or arms ■ Tense, straight arms; rigid; or rapid extension and flexion
Leg Movements 0 = Relaxed/restrained 1 = Flexed/extended	■ Relaxed, no muscle rigidity, occasional random (with soft restraints) movements of legs ■ Tense, straight legs; rigid; or rapid extension and flexion
State of Arousal 0 = Sleeping/awake 1 = Fussy	■ Quiet, peaceful, sleeping; or alert and settled ■ Alert and restless or thrashing; fussy

Note: From Lawrence, J., Alcock, D., McGrath, P., et al. (1993). The development of a tool to assess neonatal pain. *Neonatal Network, 12*(6), 61.

OUCHER SCALES

- Use in children between 3 and 7 years of age. Select the scale that matches the child's ethnic background—Caucasian, African American, or Hispanic (Figure 9-1).
- The child selects the face that matches his or her level of pain. The older child can select a number between 0 and 10.

Figure 9-1 *Oucher Pain Scale*

*In the form presented in this book, the Oucher is for educational purposes only and cannot be used for patient care.

a. Reliability is the extent to which the same score is obtained when an instrument or scale is used either by different persons or by the same person at different times. Validity is the extent to which an instrument or scale measures what it is supposed to measure.

b. (A) The Causasian version of the Oucher, developed and copyrighted by Judith E. Beyer, RN, Ph.D., 1983. (B) The African-American version of the Oucher, developed and copyrighted by Mary J. Denyes, RN, Ph.D., and Antonio M. Villarruel, RN, Ph.D., 1990. Cornelia P. Porter, RN, Ph.D. and Charlotta Marshall, RN, MSN, contributed to the development of the scale. (C) The Hispanic version of the Oucher, developed and copyrighted by Antonio M. Villarruel, RN, Ph.D., and Mary J. Denyes, RN, Ph.D., 1990. *www.oucher.org*

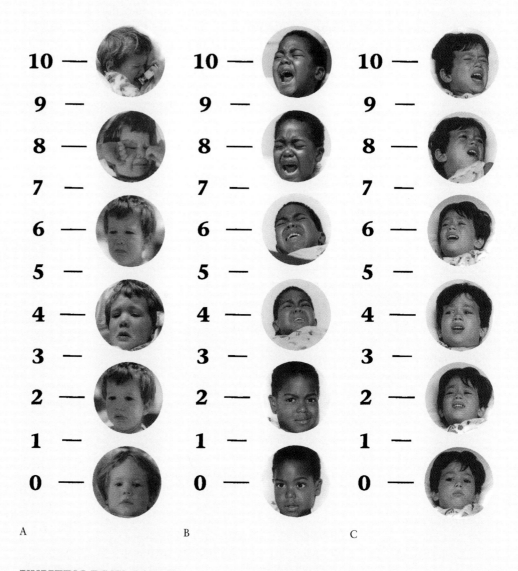

A   B   C

NUMERIC PAIN SCALE

- Use in children from 9 years to adult.
- Ask the child to rate the pain felt on a line with 10 marks, with 1 indicating a little pain and 10 indicating the most pain ever felt (Figure 9-2).

Figure 9-2 *Numeric Pain Scale*

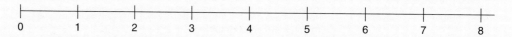

0   1   2   3   4   5   6   7   8

PREPARATION

1. Select the pain scale appropriate for the age, cooperation, and communication ability of the child.
2. Teach the cooperative and communicative child how to use the pain scale.

EQUIPMENT AND SUPPLIES

- Copy of the pain scale

PROCEDURE

1. Perform a pain assessment on a child any time an adult would be expected to have pain, such as from an injury, surgery, or illness.

   RATIONALE: *Even neonates and infants feel and remember pain. Children do not complain about pain because they fear the method to relieve pain is worse than the pain.*

2. When the child is able to verbalize, ask the child to point to the picture or number that matches the pain felt at that moment.

3. If the child has multiple injuries, ask about the pain felt at each site, and then all injuries together.

   RATIONALE: *Assessment of the pain associated with an individual injury may minimize the discomfort the child is feeling from multiple injuries.*

4. Repeat the pain assessment after analgesia is given and compare with the earlier pain assessment.

   RATIONALE: *This action determines the effectiveness of the analgesia provided.*

5. Document the pain assessment method, score, and time performed.

Special Pain Management Techniques

SKILL 9-2 Administering Patient-Controlled Analgesia (PCA) Pumps

Specially designed pumps can be used to deliver analgesia to individuals for pain control. The pumps use an intravenous line and a syringe with ordered medication is locked inside the pump. The pump is programmed so that when the patient pushes a button, an analgesic dose is administered. If it is too soon, the pump will not deliver the dose, because a lockout interval is inserted into the pump computer by the nurse. In addition, the pump can be set to administer a specific amount of medication at designated time intervals without the child pushing the button. This allows for pain control even during sleep or for young children (Figure 9-3).

PREPARATION

1. When it is assumed that a child will have patient-controlled analgesia (PCA) after surgery, bring it in before the surgery and explain its use.

   RATIONALE: *Prior explanation will enhance the child's understanding because the child is not in pain or immediately postoperative.*

2. Once ordered, check the medication order and compute the maximum 24-hour dose to verify safety.

3. Prepare the tubing and pump according to manufacturer's directions.

   RATIONALE: *The PCA tubing must be primed with IV fluid and attached with a Y connector to the IV line for the patient.*

EQUIPMENT AND SUPPLIES

- Pump
- Tubing
- IV fluid
- Medication
- Alcohol swabs

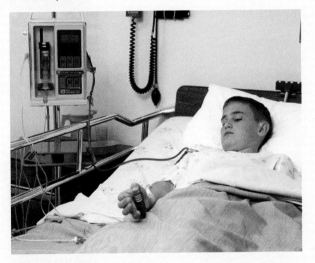

Figure 9-3 *This boy was instructed preoperatively in use of the PCA pump. Being able to administer his own analgesia when it is needed offers him a sense of control and contributes to successful pain management.*

PROCEDURE: *Clean Gloves*

1. Complete a thorough pain and physical assessment.

   RATIONALE: *Baseline data are used to evaluate pain control effectiveness and any side effects from the medication.*

2. Bring the prepared tubing, pump, and medication to the child.

3. Don gloves.
4. Attach the tubing as directed to the child's IV line.
5. Unlock the pump door and follow protocol for programming the pump delivery.
6. Deliver loading dose if ordered.
   RATIONALE: *Loading doses begin the medication process and allow pain control to be effective.*
7. Verify that the pump is locked and key is removed from room.
   RATIONALE: *Inadvertent entry of unauthorized persons into the pump mechanism must be avoided.*

SKILL 9-3 Conscious Sedation Monitoring

Conscious sedation is increasingly being used in children because it offers a method of safely performing painful procedures and avoiding trauma to the child. Consciousness is depressed while the child is able to maintain a patent airway and can respond to some verbal commands and to physical stimulation. It is important that the child who has conscious sedation be properly prepared, monitored during the procedure, and recovered after the procedure is completed.

PREPARATION

1. Inform child (if old enough to understand) and parents. Obtain informed consent.
2. Obtain assessment information (Table 9-2).
3. Evaluate recent food and fluid intake.
   RATIONALE: *Desired time to be NPO for foods is 8 hours, and for fluids the time is 4 to 6 hours.*

EQUIPMENT AND SUPPLIES

- Have drugs to be used prepared and available. Prepare emergency drugs, equipment, and personnel (Table 9-3).

   RATIONALE: *The practitioner using conscious sedation must be trained in use of the medication and in airway management. An additional support person must be present to monitor the child. All personnel present should be trained in advanced life support in emergency situations.*

- Prepare syringes and intravenous lines and fluids.
- Have respiratory suction present and functional.

TABLE 9-2	Assessments Prior to Conscious Sedation
■ Age	■ Prior reactions to sedation
■ Weight	■ Family history of diseases and anesthesia reactions
■ Height	■ Review of systems
■ Health history	■ Vital signs
■ Allergies	■ Physical examination, particularly of heart and lungs
■ Current medications	■ Psychological and developmental status
■ Diseases	■ Communication ability
■ Hospitalizations	

Note: Adapted from Bindler, R. M., & Howry, L. B. (1997). *Pediatric drugs and nursing implications* (2nd ed.). Stamford, CT: Appleton & Lange; Standards of the American Society of Anesthesiologists, House of Delegates, October 13, 1999.

TABLE 9-3 Conscious Sedation Medication

Common Medications Used for Sedation

- Chloral Hydrate
- Demerol-Phenergan-Thorazine
- Pentobarbital
- Diazepam
- Midazolam
- Morphine
- Fentanyl

Suggested Emergency Drugs

- Oxygen
- 50% glucose
- Atropine
- Epinephrine
- Phenylephrine
- Dopamine
- Diazepam
- Isoproterenol
- Calcium Chloride or Gluconate
- Sodium Bicarbonate
- Lidocaine
- Naloxone
- Diphenhydramine
- Hydrocortisone
- Succinylcholine
- Aminophylline
- Racemic epinephrine
- Inhalation albuterol
- Insulin
- Mazicon

Note: Adapted from Bindler, R. M., & Howry, L. B. (1997). *Pediatric drugs and nursing implications* (2nd ed). Stamford, CT: Appleton & Lange.

PROCEDURE: *Clean and Sterile Gloves*

During Procedure:

1. Record all drugs administered, doses, and times.
2. Monitor oxygen saturation and heart rate continuously.
3. Assess level of sedation, respiration, and blood pressure throughout the procedure.
4. Record all assessments on flowsheet.
5. Check restraints and head position throughout procedure.

After Procedure:

1. Maintain monitoring while keeping suction and emergency services available.
2. Take vital signs and complete other monitoring every 5 minutes until awake and then every 15 minutes until stable and discharged. See Table 9-4 for discharge criteria.

TABLE 9-4 Discharge Criteria from Unit After Conscious Sedation

- Satisfactory and stable cardiovascular function and airway patency.
- Easily arousable, protective reflexes intact.
- Sits up unassisted if old enough to do so.
- Discharge state is the same as admission state.
- Adequate hydration.

Note: Adapted from Bindler, R. M., & Howry, L. B. (1997). *Pediatric drugs and nursing implications* (2nd ed.). Stamford, CT: Appleton & Lange; Committee on Drugs. (1992). *Guidelines for monitoring and management of pediatric patients during and after sedation for diagnostic and therapeutic procedures.* American Academy of Pediatrics: Elk Grove Village, IL.

SKILL 9-4 Local Pain Blocks

Local pain blocks are increasingly being inserted during surgery or other procedures to offer local pain control. Commonly, microtubing is inserted into a site such as the epidural space or popliteal area, wrapped securely, and attached to an infusion pump with pain medication (Figures 9–4A and B). Local pain blocks allow the child to be alert and interactive while achieving excellent pain control.

PREPARATION

1. Have an infusion pump ready when the child may return from surgery with a local block.

2. Review the child's operative and recovery records, and the medication noted on the infusion bag.

EQUIPMENT AND SUPPLIES

- Medication and pain assessment records
- Infusion pump

PROCEDURE

1. Perform pain assessment and complete vital signs and level of consciousness.
   RATIONALE: *Baseline data will be needed for future comparison.*

2. Observe the wrapped local block site. Evaluate for swelling, redness, pallor, or leaking of solution onto bandage.

3. Monitor the infusion and maintain at ordered infusion rate (Figure 9-4C).

4. Continue to monitor regularly according to agency policy.

5. When the block is to be discontinued by the physician, provide sterile gloves, gauze pads, and tape.

6. After removal, monitor the site several times daily for 2 days for drainage or discharge.
   RATIONALE: *Continued monitoring assists in identifying infection.*

SAFETY PRECAUTIONS

The dressing around a local pain block insertion site should *not* be removed to check the site. This could inadvertently dislodge the catheter. Check the skin that is visible and the dressing for drainage, but do not remove the dressing without specific physician orders to do so.

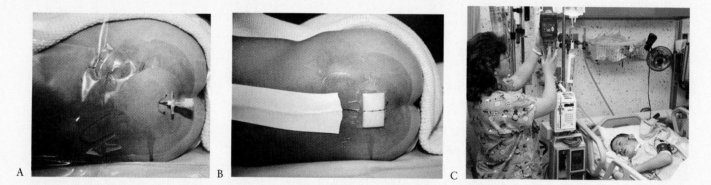

A   B   C

Figure 9-4 A, *Epidural pain block being placed during surgery and* B, *taped into place and wrapped securely.* C, *A nurse monitors the pump that is infusing pain medication into the epidural space of a boy who has had a spinal fusion. Courtesy of Shriners Hospital for Children, Spokane, WA.*

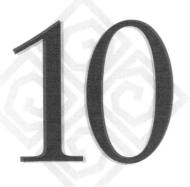

10

Cardiorespiratory Care

Chapter Outline

Administration of Oxygen

When administering oxygen, the concentration ordered and the age of the child are important. Humidification is often necessary to prevent nasal passages from drying out. Because oxygen is combustible, certain precautions must be taken during its use.

Oxygen Delivery Systems

Masks

The size of the mask is important when administering oxygen. The mask should extend from the bridge of the nose to the cleft of the chin. It should fit snugly on the face, but put no pressure on the eyes to avoid stimulating a vagal response. The following types of masks are available.

■ The *simple face mask* (Figure 10-1) can deliver from 30% to 60% oxygen when a flow rate of 6 to 10 L/min is used.

■ The *nonrebreather mask* has a reservoir bag attached to deliver higher concentrations of oxygen, from 60% to 90% with a flow of 12 to 15 L/min, when a tight seal is maintained.

Nasal Cannula

A nasal cannula is used to deliver low-flow, low-concentration oxygen. It does not provide humidified oxygen. A flow rate set higher than 6 L/min will irritate the nasopharynx without appreciably improving the child's oxygenation. The nasal cannula can deliver up to 44% oxygen with a flow rate of 1 to 6 L/min.

The prongs of the cannula are placed in the anterior nares, and the elastic band is placed around the child's head (Figure 10-2). Infants, preschool, and school-age children usually tolerate the cannula. Toddlers will usually pull the cannula off their face. A face mask or blow-by tubing is often a more appropriate method of oxygen administration for this age group.

Tent

An oxygen tent (Figure 10-3), in theory, allows for delivery of 50% humidified oxygen, but in practice only 30% humidified oxygen can be achieved. Concentration should be determined with an oxygen analyzer. To avoid air leakage, secure the edges of the tent with blankets.

Access to and visual assessment of the child is difficult when an oxygen tent is used. The child may feel confined, isolated from others, or claustrophobic when in the tent.

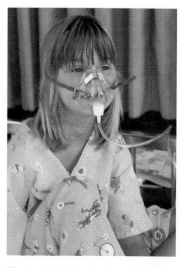

Figure 10-1 *Simple face mask.*

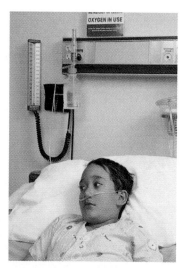

Figure 10-2 *Nasal cannula.*

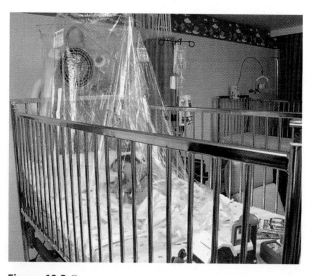

Figure 10-3 *Oxygen tent.*

The child may respond more favorably to using the mask when awake and the tent while asleep.

Blow-by Cannula

A blow-by cannula may be either a narrow oxygen catheter with small perforations through which oxygen can flow or corrugated oxygen tubing. This device is used when the child will not tolerate other means of oxygen therapy and when low oxygen concentrations with humidification are needed. The concentration of oxygen delivered varies according to the flow rate and proximity to the face. The parent can hold the child on the lap and direct the tubing toward the child's face, moving it as the child moves. This technique reduces the child's anxiety and facilitates parental involvement in care. In the ICU, the blow-by method can be used for young infants (Figure 10-4).

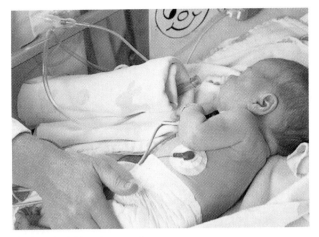

Figure 10-4 *Blow-by cannula.*

SKILL 10-1 Using Oxygen Delivery Systems

PREPARATION

1. Review the physician order for oxygen and delivery system.

2. Attach a sterile, water-filled container to the oxygen or flowmeter with a connecting tube.

3. Inform the child and parent about the need for oxygen, how it will be provided, and how they can assist with the procedure.

EQUIPMENT AND SUPPLIES

- Oxygen canister or wall outlet, tubing, and flowmeter
- Oxygen delivery system
- Sterile, water-filled container
- Oximeter

PROCEDURE

1. Perform baseline assessment of vital signs, color, respiratory effort, pulse oximetry reading, and level of consciousness.
   RATIONALE: *The baseline assessment provides comparison to measure the effectiveness of oxygen therapy.*

2. Turn on oxygen to the ordered flow rate.

3. Place the oxygen delivery device on the child's face. If the child resists the device, check the fit and try to improve the child's comfort.

4. When an oxygen tent is used, secure the edges to prevent oxygen leakage.

5. Monitor the child's response to the therapy with the previous assessments.

Cardiorespiratory Monitoring Equipment

SKILL 10-2 Oxygen Saturation: Pulse Oximetry

Pulse oximetry is a simple noninvasive method used to measure the oxygen saturation of the blood (Sao_2).

PREPARATION

1. Explain the procedure to the child and parent and why it is needed. Inform the child that pulse oximetry is a pain-free method of monitoring the oxygen level in the blood.

2. Select the appropriate sensor size for the child, either infant or pediatric sizes. Size is determined by the size of the child and/or the placement site.

3. Set the oximeter parameters for alarms according to physician directions.

EQUIPMENT AND SUPPLIES

- Pulse oximeter
- Appropriate-size sensor

PROCEDURE

1. Perform a baseline assessment before attaching the sensor. Check respiratory status, including heart rate, respiratory rate, skin color, and respiratory effort.

2. Place the sensor on the fingertip over the nail, on the toe over the nail, or on the ear lobe (Figure 10-5A and B). It should be approximately at heart level.
   RATIONALE: *The ear lobe is used when the child has poor perfusion. This is considered a central location, because a large percentage of the blood goes to the head and brain.*

3. Turn on the oximeter. Attach the sensor to the machine. Watch for readout of the pulse rate and oxygen saturation level.

4. Leave the oximeter on for continuous readouts. If frequent, but noncontinuous monitoring is ordered, leave the sensor on the child but disconnect it from the machine.
   RATIONALE: *Disconnecting the machine allows the child freedom to move and feel less confined.*

5. If the sensor is removed, place it on the plastic backing for further use.
   RATIONALE: *This practice maintains the adhesive so the sensor can be reused.*

6. Remove the sensor from the extremity at least every 2 hours to check the condition of the skin.

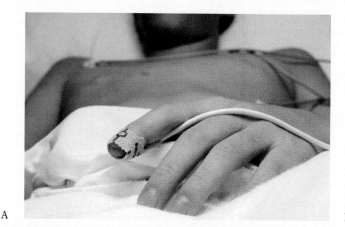
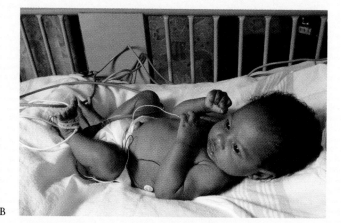

A   B

Figure 10-5 *A, Pulse oximeter on finger, and B, on foot.*

SKILL 10-3 Cardiorespiratory or Apnea Monitor

The standard cardiorespiratory monitor measures heart rate and respiratory rate when continuous assessment of the heart and respiratory rates are required. An apnea monitor is used to monitor for abnormal or irregular breathing in infants.

PREPARATION

1. Explain the procedure to the child and parents, informing them that this is a pain-free method to monitor the child's condition.

2. The high and low limits are set according to the age of the child. Usually a 15- to 20-second period of apnea will set off the alarm.

EQUIPMENT AND SUPPLIES

- Cardiorespiratory monitor
- Electrodes and straps to hold them in place
- Alcohol swabs

PROCEDURE

1. Clean the skin areas where the leads will be applied with alcohol swabs and allow to dry.

   RATIONALE: *Cleaning the skin will remove oils so the adhesive pads holding the electrodes have better adherence.*

2. Place electrodes on the child's chest: one on the right side, one on the left, and one (ground) on the lateral side of the abdomen (Figure 10-6).

3. If the monitor alarm sounds, check the child immediately. Assess breathing and heart rate.

4. If the child is not in distress, silence the alarm, check the connections and leads, and reset the alarm.

   RATIONALE: *Leads frequently become disconnected as the child moves.*

5. If the child is not breathing, stimulate the child and, if there is no response, initiate cardiopulmonary resuscitation (CPR). (See procedure later in this unit.)

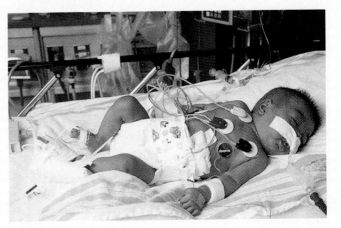

Figure 10-6 *Placement of electrodes.*

SKILL 10-4 Placement of Electrocardiogram Electrodes

The electrocardiogram is a graphic representation of the electricity produced by the heart muscle. Twelve leads are used to provide the optimal recording.

PREPARATION

1. Explain the procedure to the child and parents. Discuss the need for the child to remain still during the actual electrocardiogram.

2. Clean the sites where leads will be placed with alcohol swabs.

EQUIPMENT AND SUPPLIES

- Electrocardiogram recorder
- Patches with leads (or suction cups with conductive gel)

PROCEDURE

1. Electrodes are placed both on the chest and limbs in the locations described in Table 10-1.

   RATIONALE: *Correct placement of the electrodes is important to ensure that the electrical impulses are accurately recorded.*

2. Turn on the electrocardiogram recorder and collect the tracing.

When completed, remove the electrodes and any conductive gel with moistened gauze pads.

TABLE 10-1	Placement of Electrocardiogram Electrodes
Chest electrodes	V_1C 4th intercostal space to right of sternum
	V_2C 4th intercostal space to left of sternum
	V_3C midway between V_2 and V_4
	V_4C 5th left intercostal space at midclavicular line
	V_5C 5th left intercostal space at anterior axillary line (midway between V_4 and V_6)
	V_6C 5th left intercostal space at midaxillary line
Limb electrodes	One on each upper extremity slightly above the wrists
	One on each lower extremity just above the ankles.

SKILL 10-5 Peak Expiratory Flow Rate Monitoring

Peak expiratory flow rate (PEFR) meters are used to measure pulmonary function in children with respiratory conditions such as asthma. The PEFR meter is used frequently over a 2-week period, at different times of day to develop the child's best average reading. This best average rate is then used for comparison when the child has signs of breathing difficulty.

PREPARATION

1. Explain the procedure to the child and parents and the reasons for its use.

2. The indicator on the peak flow rate meter is placed at the bottom of the numbered scale.

3. The child's personal best score should be identified so the PEFR can be used for assessment of respiratory distress. The child's personal best is determined after reviewing the recorded PEFRs measured two to four times a day for 2 or 3 weeks. The child should be optimally treated with medications during the day so the best reading is obtained (Richmond, 1997).

4. The peak flow meter is then set to reflect the child's personal best score and "zones" indicating different levels of expiratory capacity (Table 10-2).

TABLE 10-2	Assessing Peak Expiratory Flow Rate (PEFR)	
Zone	PEFR (Best or Predicted for Age)	Action
Green	80%–100%	Continue regular management plan.
Yellow	50%–80%	An episode of asthma may be beginning. Implement action plan provided by physician.
Red	<50%	**Medical Alert:** Implement action plan predetermined by physician. Call provider if PEFR does not return to yellow or green zone.

EQUIPMENT AND SUPPLIES

- Peak flow rate meter
- Notebook to keep a log of PEFR readings

PROCEDURE

1. Have the child place the mouthpiece of the meter in the mouth (Figure 10-7). After taking a deep breath, ask the child to blow as hard and fast into the meter as possible. Read the number achieved.

2. Have the child repeat this procedure two or three more times. Average the numbers from all the readings to derive the PEFR.
   RATIONALE: *The child may need a couple of efforts to get the best reading.*

3. Compare the PEFR with the child's personal best and interpret the level of respiratory distress and the appropriate intervention.

4. Record the child's PEFR and provide medication if needed.

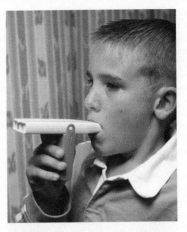

Figure 10-7 *Child using a peak flow rate meter.*

Artificial Airways

SKILL 10-6 Assisting With Oropharyngeal Airway Insertion

The oropharyngeal airway is commonly used to maintain an airway in children who are unconscious. Pediatric sizes range from 4 to 10 cm in length. The airway must be the correct size. The oropharyngeal airway is designed to keep the tongue of an unconscious child from falling into the posterior pharynx (Figure 10-8). An oropharyngeal airway is usually inserted by the physician.

PREPARATION

1. To determine the proper size airway for the child, place an airway alongside the child's face with the bite block parallel to the hard palate and the flange at the level of the central incisors. The distal end of the airway should reach the angle of the jaw (Figure 10-9). Select the airway that is the best fit for the child.
   RATIONALE: *If the airway is too large, it can obstruct the larynx. If it is too small, it will push the tongue into the posterior pharynx, causing it to obstruct the airway.*

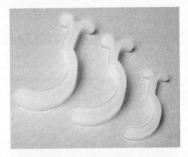

Figure 10-8 *Oropharyngeal airways of various sizes, each with flange, bite block, and curved body.*

EQUIPMENT AND SUPPLIES

- Oropharyngeal airways of different sizes
- Airway suction equipment

PROCEDURE

1. Carefully assess the child during the procedure.

2. Once the airway is in place, maintain the child's head and jaw in a neutral position, neither flexed forward nor extended.
   RATIONALE: *This position keeps the trachea from being crimped.*

3. If the child regains consciousness, remove the oropharyngeal airway.
   RATIONALE: *The airway will stimulate the gag reflex and vomiting that can increase the risk for aspiration.*

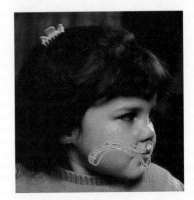

Figure 10-9 *Estimating the size of an oropharyngeal airway.*

SKILL 10-7 Assisting With Nasopharyngeal Airway Insertion

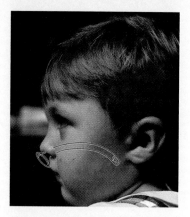

Figure 10-10 *Estimating the size of a nasopharyngeal airway.*

The nasopharyngeal airway provides a passage for air between the tongue and the posterior pharyngeal wall. It is used for a conscious child with an obstructed airway, or a child who potentially may lose consciousness and lose an open airway. The airway is made of soft plastic or rubber and comes in various sizes. The airway must be the correct size. The physician usually inserts the airway in a posterior direction.

PREPARATION

1. Select the correct size nasopharyngeal airway. The length of the tube is determined by measuring the distance from the tip of the nose to the tragus of the ear (Figure 10-10). The width must allow for passage through the nares.

2. Explain the procedure to the child and parents. Tell them not to touch the airway to prevent it from being dislodged.

3. Lubricate the tip with water-soluble gel.

EQUIPMENT AND SUPPLIES

- Nasopharyngeal airways of different sizes
- Water-soluble lubricant

PROCEDURE

1. Observe for bleeding in the back of the throat. Blood may exacerbate the obstruction and further compromise airway management.
   RATIONALE: *Insertion of the tube may cause trauma to the nasopharyngeal airway passage.*

2. Assess the child's respiratory rate and effort.

SKILL 10-8 Tracheostomy General Guidelines

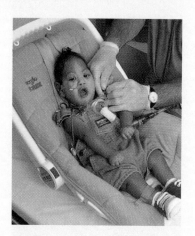

Figure 10-11 *Infant with a tracheostomy collar.*

A tracheostomy is a surgical procedure in which an opening is made through the neck into the trachea to create an airway. It may be performed by a physician as an acute life-saving procedure or for management of the child with a chronic disease.

A neonatal or pediatric *tracheostomy tube* is made of plastic and has an obturator used for insertion only. The tube is held in place with twill tape tied around the child's neck. The child usually wears a *tracheostomy collar* (Figure 10-11) (mist collar) at the stoma site to keep the airway warm and moist. The collar may emit either oxygen or room air, depending on the physician's orders.

PREPARATION

1. When a child with a tracheostomy is admitted, plan for close monitoring of the child's respiratory status.

2. Obtain equipment and supplies for any emergency intervention needed.

EQUIPMENT AND SUPPLIES

- Resuscitation bag
- Oxygen
- Suctioning equipment
- Tracheostomy tubes, one the size of the child's current tube and one a size smaller
- Twill tape

PROCEDURE

1. Carefully observe the child with a tracheostomy for signs of obstruction.

2. Vital signs and respiratory status, including breath sounds, respiratory effort, and airway patency, should be routinely checked. Be alert for changes in heart or respiratory rate, blood pressure, color, or level of consciousness.

3. Watch for condensation in the oxygen tubing and empty it regularly.

    RATIONALE: *Fluid may drip into the tracheostomy tube, causing the child to aspirate if the oxygen tubing is not emptied regularly.*

4. When the child is in a crib, put the tubing through, rather than over, the bars.

    RATIONALE: *This prevents fluid from entering the tracheostomy.*

SKILL 10-9 Tracheostomy Care

Tracheostomy care is usually performed once per shift. An assistant should *always* be present while tracheostomy care is being performed.

PREPARATION

1. Have an assistant stand on the opposite side of the bed.

2. Prepared tracheostomy tubes, oxygen, resuscitation bag, and suction tray with catheters should be at bedside.

3. Prepare new ties for the tracheostomy tube. Cut two pieces of twill tape, about 12 in. each. Fold one end of each piece over lengthwise for approximately 1 to 1.5 in. Cut a small hole in the folded end.

4. Place a towel roll under the child's neck to hyperextend it.

    RATIONALE: *Hyperextension will provide greater access to the neck, especially in infants and young children who have such short necks.*

EQUIPMENT AND SUPPLIES

- Towel roll
- Precut twill tape
- Cotton-tipped applicators saturated with half-strength hydrogen peroxide
- Cotton-tipped applicators saturated with normal saline
- Gauze pads (some moistened with saline and others dry)
- Scissors
- Tracheal cleaning tray with sterile bowls, pipe cleaners, brush, notched gauze pad
- Sterile hydrogen peroxide and sterile normal saline
- Suction tray and catheters

Note: Equipment is usually available in a prepackaged kit.

PROCEDURE: *Sterile Gloves*

1. Don sterile gloves.

2. Pour sterile normal saline into a sterile bowl and hydrogen peroxide into another bowl.

3. Unlock the inner cannula and place it into the bowl containing the hydrogen peroxide. Clean the cannula thoroughly with pipe cleaners and rinse in normal saline. Replace the inner cannula and lock it into place.

    RATIONALE: *The inner cannula becomes obstructed with airway secretions and must be cleaned regularly to keep the airway open.*

4. Using cotton-tipped applicators saturated with half-strength hydrogen peroxide, clean under the tracheostomy tube at the stoma site (Figure 10-12). With the tapes still tied, rinse the stoma with saline applicators. Wash the area behind the flanges of the tracheostomy and around the neck with damp gauze, observing for redness or skin breakdown. Dry thoroughly.

    RATIONALE: *The airway secretions irritate the skin and cause skin breakdown if not removed regularly.*

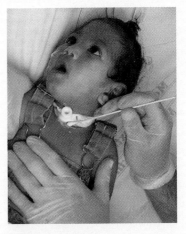

Figure 10-12 *Cleaning the tracheostomy tube.*

5. Hold the tube while an assistant performs the same care on the opposite side.

6. Place a notched gauze pad under the stoma.

7. To replace the ties for the tube, have the assistant hold the tube in place. Cut the tapes and remove the old ties from the flange of the tube.

   RATIONALE: *This practice prevents the tube from being expelled if the child coughs or moves unexpectedly.*

8. Attach the twill tape to the flange by first threading the end with the slit through the hole. Place the distal end of the twill tape through the slit and pull it securely.

9. Have the assistant repeat this step on the opposite side while you hold the tube in place.

10. With the tube held in place, tie the tape. The best fit is achieved when the child's neck is slightly flexed. The tape should be tied tightly enough to prevent dislodgment but should still be loose enough so that you can fit one finger between it and the child's neck.

11. Double- or triple-knot the tape for security. Place the knot at the side of the child's neck.

    RATIONALE: *Having the knot on the side prevents skin irritation when the child is supine.*

SKILL 10-10 Endotracheal Tube Care

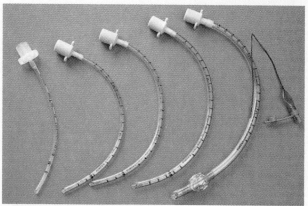

Figure 10-13 *Endotracheal tubes.*

An endotracheal (ET) tube is an emergency artificial airway used to maintain and secure an open airway in an unconscious child. ET tubes are sterile, disposable, and made of a translucent plastic or other synthetic material. The distal end is tapered and has an opening in the side wall (Murphy's eye). The length of the tube is marked in centimeters to serve as a measurement reference point once it is in place. The tubes come in various sizes, both with and without cuffs (Figure 10-13). The uncuffed tube is recommended for the child younger than 8 or 9 years, because the airway is narrowest at the cricoid ring, sealing the airway effectively without a cuff.

PREPARATION

1. Select the appropriate size tube for the child. Use a length-based resuscitation tape or formula to select tube size (see Table 10-3). The size of the tube can be approximated by comparing it with the diameter of the child's fingernail on the fifth finger. The formula used for children older than 2 years is as follows:

$$(16 + \text{Age in years}) \div 4 = \text{Size of ET tube}$$

2. Position the child in supine position with neck hyperextended.

EQUIPMENT AND SUPPLIES

- Endotracheal tubes of different sizes, cuffed and uncuffed
- Pediatric stylet
- Length-based resuscitation tape
- Tape
- Larynoscope with curved and straight blades of different sizes
- Water-soluble lubricant
- Resuscitation bag
- Suction catheter

PROCEDURE

1. Intubation is usually performed by the physician or paramedic to protect or maintain the child's airway. The tube is held in position until taped securely.

   RATIONALE: *The position of the tube can easily shift with movement of the child's head and neck. Correct placement of the tube in the trachea is critical for survival of the child.*

TABLE 10-3	Suggested Endotracheal Tube and Suction Catheter Sizes	
Age	Endotracheal Tube Size (mm)	Suction Catheter Size (French)
Premature newborn	2.0–2.5	5
Newborn	3.0–3.5	6–8
6 months	3.5	8
12–18 months	4.0	8
3 years	4.5	8
5 years	5.0	10
6 years	5.5	10
8 years	6.0	10
12 years	6.5	10
16 years	7.0–8.0	12

Note: *Adapted from Dieckman, R., Brownstein, D., & Gaushe-Hill, M. (eds.). (2000). Pediatric education for prehospital professionals/American Academy of Pediatrics. Sudbury, MA: Jones and Bartlett Publishers.*

2. Once the tube has been placed by the physician, auscultate for equal breath sounds, and check for symmetry of chest movement and condensation in the tube. Auscultate over the abdomen for any bubbling or gurgling sounds to ensure that the tube is not in the esophagus. Listen at the trachea for air leaks.

3. Once correct tube placement is verified, note the centimeter marking at the lip or tooth line and tape the tube in place.

    RATIONALE: *Placing a mark on the tube provides a quick method of confirming placement of the tube during future assessments.*

4. Reassess tube placement after the tube is taped.

5. Continuously assess breath sounds, color, heart rate on the monitor, and pulse oximeter readout.

    RATIONALE: *The child with an endotracheal tube needs constant assessment to ensure that the tube does not become dislodged from the trachea.*

6. Initiate assisted ventilation if spontaneous breathing is not present.

Assisted Ventilation

SKILL 10-11 Bag-Valve-Mask Ventilation

Resuscitation bags and masks are used to perform assisted ventilation for the child who is unable to breathe adequately on his or her own. This is an emergency procedure, performed until airway control is attained and a ventilator is provided.

PREPARATION

1. Select the appropriate-size mask for the child. The mask should extend from the bridge of the nose to the cleft of the chin (Figure 10–14). The correct size mask has a small volume that minimizes dead space and prevents rebreathing of expired carbon dioxide.

2. Select the appropriate-size resuscitation bag for the child. The pediatric bag should have a volume of 450 to 750 mL. An adult bag (1,200 mL) can be used with older children.

    RATIONALE: *Pediatric tidal volume is approximately 8 mL/kg. The bag size should be no smaller than the child's tidal volume.*

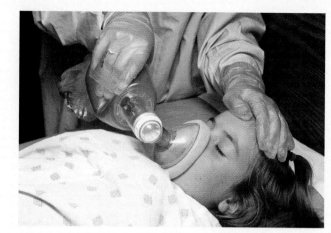

Figure 10-14 *Bag-valve-mask ventilation.*

3. Connect the oxygen tubing to the resuscitation bag, and to the flowmeter. Set the oxygen flow to 15 L/min.

4. If the resuscitation bag has a pop-off valve, block it.
   RATIONALE: *This allows higher inspiratory pressures to be achieved when used to ensure chest rise.*

EQUIPMENT AND SUPPLIES

- Self-inflating resuscitation bag and mask
- Oxygen and tubing
- Suction and appropriate-size catheters
- Pulse oximeter
- Oropharyngeal or nasopharyngeal airway

PROCEDURE: *Clean Gloves*

1. Assess the child's respiratory status and initiate assisted ventilation when the child is unable to breathe at an adequate rate.

2. Open the child's airway with a head-tilt/chin-lift or jaw thrust maneuver. (See CPR section later in this chapter.) Use an oropharyngeal or nasopharyngeal airway if airway patency cannot be maintained.

3. Place a towel roll under the infant's or toddler's shoulders to achieve a sniffing position. Avoid hyperextending the neck.
   RATIONALE: *The head of the infant and toddler is large, and lifting the shoulders places the airway in a neutral position.*

4. Apply the mask to the face and get an airtight seal. Pull the child's jaw into the mask rather than pushing the mask into the face. Use an assistant to maintain the seal.
   RATIONALE: *Failure to achieve a seal will result in a lower oxygen concentration or inadequate volume of air.*

5. Begin ventilation by squeezing the bag. Watch for chest rise. Squeeze the bag only until the chest rise is visible, then release.
   RATIONALE: *Using more force than needed to make the chest rise will push air into the stomach and potentially cause the child to vomit, compromising the airway.*

6. With each ventilation, say "squeeze, release, release." The rate of ventilation should be 30/min in infants and 20/min in children.
   RATIONALE: *The child needs a 1:2 inspiratory to expiratory ratio and this phrase provides a reminder.*

7. Assess the effectiveness of ventilations by observing for bilateral chest rise, auscultating lung sounds, and monitoring pulse oximeter level.

SKILL 10-12 Ventilator

Ventilators are used for children who need assistance with breathing. These children may have a chronic condition, such as a neuromuscular disease or persistent lung pathology, or may be acutely ill or injured and need emergency management of ventilation. The ventilator is usually attached to the child's endotracheal tube or tracheostomy tube.

PREPARATION

1. Become familiar with the ventilator and know the settings ordered by the physician (oxygen concentration, humidity, air temperature, pressure, tidal volume, and inspiratory/expiratory ratio and rate). Identify what the alarms mean, and know how to troubleshoot problems.

EQUIPMENT AND SUPPLIES

- Ventilator
- Cardiorespiratory monitor

- Pulse oximeter
- Resuscitation bag and mask
- Suction and appropriate-size catheters
- Oxygen
- Nasogastric tube

PROCEDURE

1. Ensure that the child is attached to a cardiorespiratory monitor and pulse oximeter.

2. Measure arterial blood gases within 15 minutes after the child has been placed on the ventilator, and thereafter according to the physician's orders.

3. Assess vital signs every hour, including heart and respiratory rates, blood pressure, temperature, and pulse oximeter reading. Auscultate the lungs in all fields to assess for equal breath sounds. Ensure that the child's respiratory rate is consistent with the ventilator setting.

4. An orogastric or nasogastric tube may be inserted.
   RATIONALE: *The tube keeps the stomach decompressed to prevent the child from vomiting and compromising the airway.*

5. Suction the endotracheal tube or tracheostomy tube as necessary (see section later in this chapter).

6. Protect the endotracheal tube by making sure it is well taped and secure. Support the ventilator tubing to decrease traction on the endotracheal tube by attaching the tubing directly to the bed using a gauze roll and a safety pin.

7. Carefully monitor the child to determine if elbow restraints are needed to prevent dislodgement of the endotracheal tube. Acutely ill or injured children may be chemically paralyzed and sedated while on the ventilator. If the child has been given paralytics, watch for signs that further sedation may be needed (e.g., a rise in heart rate and blood pressure or tearing).

8. Listen and look for air leaks. Make sure that the ventilator is firmly attached to the endotracheal tube or tracheostomy tube.

9. Check the reservoir for humidification at least every 8 hours. Refill or replace water as needed. Watch for condensation in the tubing and empty it regularly.
   RATIONALE: *If fluid is not removed from the tubing, it may drip into the endotracheal tube, causing the child to aspirate.*

10. Explain the procedure to the child. For example: "I am going to wash your face" or "I am going to move your arms and legs." The child who is sedated or unresponsive may still be able to hear.

11. Support the family by answering questions. Encourage family members to talk to the child and to bring in audiotapes of favorite music or of others speaking to the child.

Cardiopulmonary Resuscitation

Cardiopulmonary resuscitation (CPR) is basic life support using techniques to maintain airway, breathing, and circulation (the ABCs). Laypeople are routinely taught one-person basic life support. Health care professionals should be skilled in both one- and two-person CPR.

SKILL 10-13 Performing Cardiopulmonary Resuscitation

PREPARATION

1. Become certified in basic life support and maintain certification.
2. Assess the child for unresponsiveness, lack of breathing, and no heart rate.
3. Call for help.

EQUIPMENT AND SUPPLIES
- Resuscitation bag and mask
- Pocket mask

PROCEDURE: *Clean Gloves*
Infant

1. Determine unresponsiveness by gently tapping the infant on the abdomen or soles of the feet. If the infant does not respond, begin basic life support (BLS) after calling for help.

2. Position the infant on the back while supporting the head and neck.

3. Open the airway by performing a chin lift: Tilt the head back and lift the chin up and out. An alternate procedure for opening the airway on an infant suspected of having a cervical spine injury is a jaw thrust: From behind the infant's head, place two or three fingers under each side of the jaw at its angle and lift the jaw upward and outward (Figure 10-15 and 10-16).

4. Look, listen, and feel for breathing. Check for the rise and fall of the chest and abdomen, and listen and feel for the flow of expelled air at the mouth (Figure 10-17).

5. Begin rescue breathing if no spontaneous breathing is detected. Seal your lips or a pocket mask tightly around the infant's mouth and nose. Maintain airway patency with the chin lift or jaw thrust maneuver. Give two slow breaths (1 to 1.5 sec), just until the chest rises (Figure 10-18). **RATIONALE:** *Slow breaths reduce the pressure that could damage the alveoli during inspiration.*

6. If the chest does not rise, check the child's position with the chin lift or jaw thrust, and repeat the two slow breaths. If the chest still does not rise, perform the procedure for choking later in this unit.

CLINICAL TIP

Gastric distention can occur with either mouth-to-mouth or resuscitation bag and mask rescue breathing. This distention compromises ventilation by elevating the diaphragm and decreasing lung size. It may also stimulate vomiting.

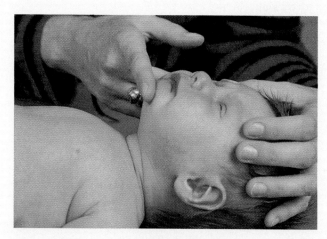

Figure 10-15 *Head tilt–chin lift maneuver.*

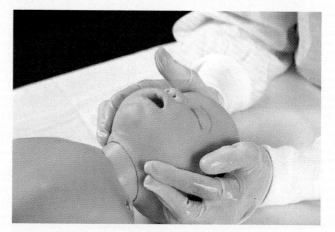

Figure 10-16 *Jaw thrust maneuver.*

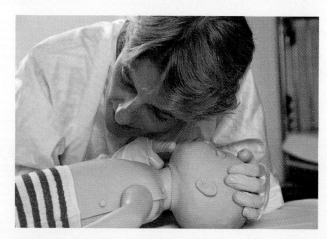

Figure 10-17 *Assessing breathing.*

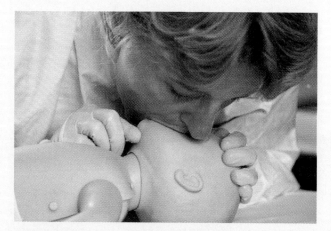

Figure 10-18 *Mouth-to-mouth-and-nose resuscitation.*

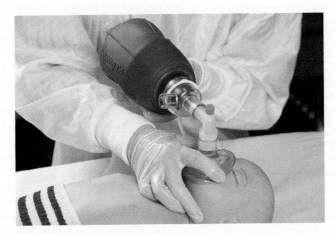

Figure 10-19 *Bag and mask resuscitation.*

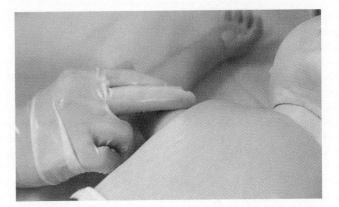

Figure 10-20 *Checking for the brachial pulse.*

7. Convert to a resuscitation bag and mask hooked up to 100% oxygen as soon as possible (Figure 10–19). Continue rescue breathing for as long as the child is not breathing. Continue slow breaths, just until the chest rises.

   RATIONALE: *More forceful breaths force excess air volume into the stomach.*

8. If the chest rises with rescue breathing, assess for signs of circulation before beginning chest compressions. Check the brachial pulse for 10 seconds before determining pulselessness (Figure 10-20).

9. If there are signs of circulation, give one slow breath every 3 seconds for 1 minute (20 breaths per minute) while keeping the airway open.

10. If there are no signs of circulation, begin chest compressions. Find the finger position near the lower half of the breastbone, making sure fingers are not over the xiphoid process (Figure 10-21).

    RATIONALE: *Pressure on the xiphoid may cause injury to underlying organs.*

11. Perform 5 compressions and 1 breath at a rate that provides 100 compressions and 20 breaths per minutes. The compression depth is 0.5 to 1 in.

12. Reassess the infant after 20 cycles (one "CPR minute"). Palpate the brachial pulse for 5 seconds. If the pulse is absent, continue the cycle for another 3 to 5 minutes before reassessment.

13. Repeat the cycle of five compressions and one breath until signs of circulation return or until help arrives.

14. If the infant has a return of both pulse and respirations and is *not* a trauma victim, place the infant in the side-lying position to protect the airway.

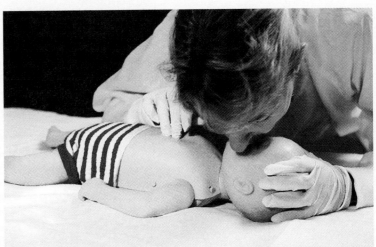

Figure 10-21 *Alternating breathing and chest compressions.*

PROCEDURE: *Clean Gloves*

Child Between 1 and 8 Years

1. Determine unresponsiveness by stimulating the child, and boldly ask "Are you all right?" If the child does not respond, call for help and begin BLS.

2. Position the child on the back while supporting the head and neck. If a head or neck injury is suspected, do not bend or turn the neck.

3. Open the airway by performing a chin lift: Tilt the head back and lift the chin up and out. An alternate procedure for opening the airway on a child suspected of having a cervical spine injury is a jaw thrust: From behind the child's head, place two or three fingers under each side of the jaw at its angle and lift the jaw upward and outward.

4. Look, listen, and feel for breathing. Check for the rise and fall of the chest and abdomen, and listen and feel for the flow of expelled air at the mouth.

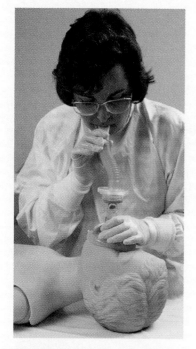

Figure 10-22 *Mouth-to-mouth resuscitation using a mask with a one-way valve.*

5. Begin rescue breathing if no spontaneous breathing is detected. Seal your lips or a pocket mask tightly around the child's mouth. Pinch the nose shut. Maintain airway patency with the chin lift or jaw thrust maneuver. Give two slow breaths (1 to 1.5 sec), just until the chest rises (Figure 10-22).

6. If the chest does not rise, check the child's position with the chin lift or jaw thrust, and repeat the two slow breaths. If the chest still does not rise, perform the procedure for choking described later in this unit.

   RATIONALE: *The child could have an airway obstruction.*

7. Convert to a resuscitation bag and mask hooked up to 100% oxygen as soon as possible. Ensure that the mask is the correct size, extending from the bridge of the nose to the cleft of the chin, but not covering the eyes. Continue rescue breathing for as long as the child is not breathing.

   RATIONALE: *Pressure on the eyes stimulates a vagal response, and thus a slowed heart rate. This must be avoided because the child is already compromised.*

8. If the chest rises with rescue breathing, assess for signs of circulation before beginning chest compressions. Check the carotid pulse for 10 seconds before determining pulselessness (Figure 10-23).

9. If there are signs of circulation, give one slow breath every 3 seconds for 1 minute (20 breaths per minute) while keeping the airway open. Continue as long as the child is not breathing spontaneously.

10. If there are no signs of circulation, begin chest compressions. Place the heel of one hand on the lower half of the breastbone. Make sure the hand is not over the xiphoid process (Figure 10-24). The compression depth is 1.0 to 1.5 in.

11. At the end of each compression, allow the chest to return to the normal position before beginning the next compression. Maintain the head tilt.

    RATIONALE: *It is important to keep the head positioned so that airway patency is maintained.*

12. Perform cycles of 5 compressions and 1 breath at a rate that provides 100 compressions and 20 breaths per minutes.

13. Reassess the child after 20 cycles (one "CPR minute"). Palpate the carotid pulse for 5 seconds. If the pulse is absent, continue the cycle for another 3 to 5 minutes before reassessment. A brief pause may also be taken for rescuers to change position.

14. Repeat the cycle of five compressions and one breath until signs of circulation return.

15. If the child has a return of both pulse and respirations and is *not* a trauma victim, place the child in the side-lying position.

    RATIONALE: *This position is used to protect the airway.*

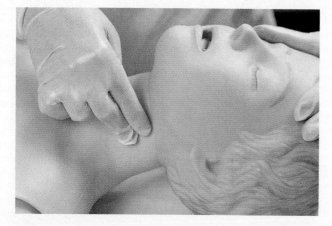

Figure 10-23 *Checking for the carotid pulse.*

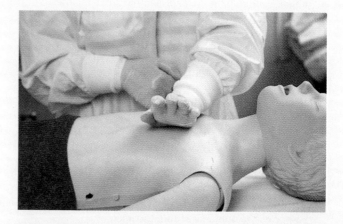

Figure 10-24 *Hand position for chest compressions.*

Foreign Body Airway Obstruction

An airway obstruction may be caused by respiratory disorders (e.g., croup or epiglottitis) or a foreign body. Attempts to clear the airway should be made in the following situations: for the witnessed or strongly suspected aspiration of a foreign body or when the airway remains obstructed during attempts to provide rescue breathing.

SKILL 10-14 Removing a Foreign Body Airway Obstruction

PREPARATION

1. When the infant or child is suspected of aspirating, encourage the child to continue crying or coughing and breathing as long as the cough is forceful. Call emergency medical services and try to keep the child calm.

   RATIONALE: *Emergency care should be sought because the infant or child may develop a complete obstruction.*

2. If the cough becomes ineffective and soundless, if increased respiratory difficulty or stridor is noted, or if the victim loses consciousness, attempts must be made to remove the obstruction.

3. If an infant is found unconscious, assess by using the ABCs (airway, breathing, and circulation). If the infant is not breathing, call aloud for help.

EQUIPMENT AND SUPPLIES

- Pocket mask

PROCEDURE: *Clean Gloves*

Infant

1. If the infant is not breathing, try to ventilate either by mouth-to-mouth resuscitation or with a bag and mask (refer to the CPR guidelines for rescue breathing). If the airway is obstructed, reposition the infant's head and attempt to ventilate again.

2. Position the infant face down on your arm supporting the head.

3. Perform five back blows with the heel of the hand between the infant's shoulder blades (Figure 10-25).

4. Position the infant face up on your forearm. Place the fingers in the same position used for CPR (Figure 10-26). Give five chest thrusts near the center of the breastbone.

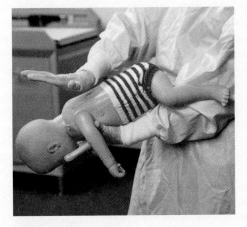

Figure 10-25 *Back blows.*

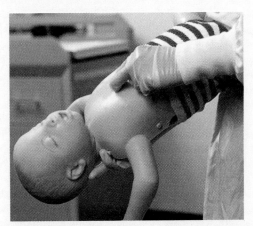

Figure 10-26 *Chest thrusts.*

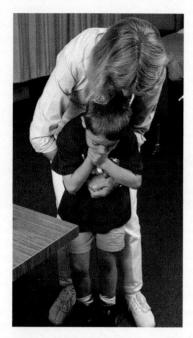

Figure 10-27 *Abdominal thrusts (Heimlich maneuver).*

5. Place your index finger on the bony prominence of the infant's chin and your thumb in the mouth on the tongue. Pull up and out to open the mouth. Look in the infant's mouth for the foreign body and remove it if seen. Do not perform a blind sweep.
   RATIONALE: *A blind sweep may actually push an obstruction deeper into the trachea.*

6. If no object is found, try to ventilate the infant again. If the obstruction is still present, reposition the infant's head and attempt to ventilate once again.

7. If the obstruction remains, begin another series of back blows and chest thrusts. Look in the mouth, try to ventilate, reposition the head, and attempt to ventilate again. Continue with this pattern until the airway is clear.

8. If the infant becomes unconscious, begin the CPR guidelines described earlier in this unit.

9. Once the airway is clear, give two slow full breaths. Check for a pulse. At this point, provide whatever BLS maneuvers are necessary.

PROCEDURE: *Clean Gloves*

Child Between 1 and 8 Years

Conscious Child

1. Perform abdominal thrusts (Heimlich maneuver) on the child in either a sitting or standing position (Figure 10-27).

2. Stand behind the child, with your arms under the child's axilla and around the chest. Place the thumb of one fist against the abdomen in the midline, below the xiphoid and above the navel. Grasp your fist with your other hand.
   RATIONALE: *Avoid the xiphoid to prevent injury to underlying organs.*

3. Deliver up to five quick upward thrusts. Each thrust should be a distinct effort to remove the obstruction.

4. The series of five thrusts should be repeated until the obstruction is cleared or the child becomes unconscious. If the child become unconscious, progress to the procedure for the unconscious child.
   RATIONALE: *Once unconscious, move the child to the floor to prevent injury and provide leverage for abdominal thrusts.*

Unconscious Child

1. Assess for breathing. If the child is not breathing, try to ventilate either by mouth-to-mouth resuscitation or with a bag and mask (refer to the CPR guidelines for rescue breathing presented earlier in this unit). If the airway is obstructed, reposition the child's head and attempt to ventilate again.

2. Place the child in a supine position and kneel, straddling the child's body at the hips and facing the child's head.
   RATIONALE: *This position makes it easier to provide the upward abdominal thrusts.*

3. Place the heel of your hand on the child's abdomen in the midline, between the xiphoid and navel; then place your other hand over the wrist (Figure 10-28). Press into the abdomen, using both hands in quick upward strokes.

4. Deliver up to five thrusts. Each thrust should be a distinct attempt to eliminate the obstruction.

5. Using the tongue–jaw lift described earlier for the unconscious infant, look into the mouth for a foreign body and remove it if seen. Do not perform a blind sweep.

6. If a foreign body is not visualized, open the airway and attempt to ventilate. If the airway is still obstructed, reposition the child's head and attempt to ventilate once again.
   RATIONALE: *The obstruction may have moved enough to permit a small airway opening.*

7. If the obstruction remains, begin another series of abdominal thrusts, look in the mouth, try to ventilate, reposition the head, and attempt to ventilate again. Continue with this process until the airway is clear.

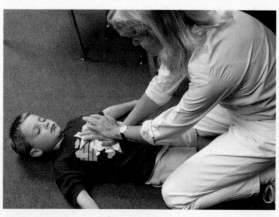

Figure 10-28 *Performing abdominal thrusts on an unconscious child.*

8. Once the airway is clear, give two slow full breaths. Check for a pulse. At this point, provide whatever BLS maneuvers are necessary.

Suctioning

Suctioning of the airway is needed when excess secretions are present or when a decreased level of consciousness interferes with the child's ability to clear normal secretions. Suctioning of the nose, mouth, tracheostomy tube, or endotracheal tube may be performed. The size of the suction catheter depends on the size, age, and weight of the child or on the tube requiring suctioning.

Nasal/Oral Suctioning

A bulb syringe is used to remove secretions from an infant's nose or mouth. A tonsil-tip or Yankauer catheter may be used for oral suctioning in children when copious, thick secretions or emesis must be removed.

SKILL 10-15 Performing Nasal/Oral Suctioning

PREPARATION

1. Assess the child's respiratory status, including breath sounds, respiratory effort, and airway patency. Observe for excess secretions that the child is unable to manage by swallowing.

2. An assistant may be needed to gently hold the child and keep the child's hands out of the way. The child's head should be maintained in the midline position.

3. Turn on and set the wall suction to the pressure level ordered by the physician or suggested in the facility's procedure manual.

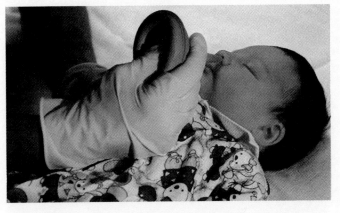

EQUIPMENT AND SUPPLIES

- Bulb syringe
- Normal saline nose drops
- Yankauer or tonsil-tip suction catheter
- Normal saline solution

PROCEDURE: *Clean Gloves*

Bulb Syringe

1. Place saline nose drops in the naris.
   RATIONALE: *The nose drops loosen dried secretions.*

2. Deflate the bulb. Insert the tip of the bulb syringe into the infant's naris (Figure 10-29).
   RATIONALE: *Deflating the bulb first prevents pushing the secretions back into the nasopharynx.*

3. Release the bulb and remove the syringe from the naris (Figure 10-30). Expel the secretions into the proper receptacle.

4. Assess the child's ability to breathe easily. Repeat the suctioning as necessary.

PROCEDURE: *Clean Gloves*

Yankauer

1. Insert catheter tip into the mouth and turn on suction.

2. Suction to remove secretions from the mouth and pharynx. Avoid causing a gag reflex.
   RATIONALE: *The gag reflex may stimulate vomiting and compromise the airway.*

3. Rinse the catheter with normal saline.

4. Assess the child's respiratory status. Repeat suctioning if needed.

Figure 10-29 *Insertion of a deflated bulb syringe.*

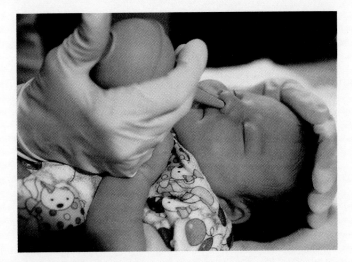

Figure 10-30 *Removal of a reinflated bulb syringe.*

SKILL 10-16 Suctioning a Conscious (Awake and Alert) Child

A catheter is used to remove secretions from an older child's mouth or nose, a tracheostomy tube, or an endotracheal tube. The child with a decreased level of consciousness will likely require deep suctioning to remove secretions (see next section).

PREPARATION

1. Have an assistant help maintain the child's head in the midline position and hold the hands out of the way. Raise the head of the bed to 30 to 45 degrees.

2. Turn on and set the wall suction to the pressure level ordered by the physician or suggested in the facility's procedure manual.

3. Attach the proximal end of the catheter to the wall suction connecting tubing, making sure to keep the distal end sterile.

EQUIPMENT AND SUPPLIES

- Appropriate-size suction catheter
- Sterile container with sterile normal saline
- Suction kit
- Water-soluble lubricant

PROCEDURE: *Sterile Gloves*

1. Keep your dominant hand sterile and your nondominant hand clean for the procedure.

2. With your dominant hand, insert the suction catheter into the child's naris and suction for no more than 5 to 10 seconds, while gently rotating the catheter. (The depth of insertion depends on the size of the child.)

NOTE: The mouth may also be suctioned for secretions, but care must be taken to avoid stimulating the gag reflex.

> RATIONALE: *Suctioning longer than 10 seconds causes vagal stimulation and bradycardia.*

3. Remove and irrigate the catheter with sterile normal saline.

4. Assess the child's respiratory status and repeat as necessary.

SKILL 10-17 Suctioning a Child with Decreased Level of Consciousness

The child with decreased level of consciousness is unable to get the secretions higher up into airway. Therefore, deeper suction is often needed to clear the airway.

PREPARATION

An assistant may be needed to keep the child's head in the midline position.

1. Raise the head of the bed to 30 to 45 degrees.

2. Turn on and set the wall suction to the pressure level ordered by the physician or suggested in the facility's procedure manual.

3. Attach the proximal end of the catheter to the wall suction connecting tubing, making sure to keep the distal end sterile.

EQUIPMENT AND SUPPLIES

- Appropriate-size suction catheter (See Table 10-3 on page 97)
- Sterile container with sterile normal saline

- Resuscitation bag and mask
- Oxygen

PROCEDURE: *Sterile Gloves*

1. Place an oxygen mask on the child's face.
   RATIONALE: *Because suctioning potentially causes hypoxia, oxygenate the child prior to suctioning.*

2. If possible, encourage the child to cough to make the secretions pool in the hypopharynx.
   RATIONALE: *This step may prevent the need for deep suctioning.*

3. Keep your dominant hand sterile and your nondominant hand clean for the procedure. Use only the dominant hand to manipulate the catheter.

4. Remove the protective sheath from the catheter, and test the suction by placing it in a cup of saline.

5. Remove the child's oxygen mask.

6. For *nasal/oral* suctioning, use your dominant hand to insert the catheter into the child's naris or mouth without occluding the suction port.
   RATIONALE: *This decreases the time of suctioning and reduces the risk for hypoxia.*

7. Slowly advance the catheter only into the hypopharynx. Occlude the suction port and rotate the catheter, applying intermittent suction for 5 to 10 seconds.

8. Remove the catheter and clear the tubing with sterile saline. Repeat as necessary.

9. For *deep suctioning,* use your dominant hand to insert the catheter (without occluding the suction port) beyond the hypopharynx and into the trachea (the length advanced is determined by the size of the child).

10. When the catheter is in place, gently rotate it while suctioning intermittently. To prevent hypoxia, do not suction for more than 5 to 10 seconds.
    RATIONALE: *Rotating the catheter ensures that the catheter eye has the greatest access to secretions.*

11. Remove the catheter and clear the tubing with sterile saline. Repeat as necessary.

12. Allow the child to breath normally, and give supplemental oxygen between suctionings.
    RATIONALE: *Because of the risk for hypoxia and bradycardia, give oxygen to improve oxygen status.*

SKILL 10-18 Tracheostomy Tube Suctioning

A tracheostomy is an opening through the neck directly into the trachea. It is used to provide adequate ventilation when the child is unable to breathe effectively alone. This opening is performed surgically and must be treated carefully to maintain patency, ensure freedom from infection, and promote adequate oxygenation.

PREPARATION

1. An assistant may be needed to hold the child and keep hands out of the way.

2. Place the head of the bed at a 30-degree angle.

3. Turn on and set the wall suction to the pressure level ordered by the physician or suggested in the facility's procedure manual.

4. Turn on the oxygen source attached to the resuscitation bag to inflate the reservoir bag so it is ready to use.

5. Attach the proximal end of the catheter to the wall suction connecting tubing, making sure to keep the distal end sterile.

EQUIPMENT AND SUPPLIES

- Additional prepared tracheostomy tubes (see earlier description on tracheostomy care)
- Resuscitation bag with attached oxygen source

CLINICAL TIP

Obtain baseline vital signs before and after the procedure. When suctioning, watch for a decrease in pulse rate, an increase or decrease in respiratory rate, or a change in color. Bradycardia may be a sign of vagal stimulation. If any of these signs occur, stop immediately and give the child oxygen using blow-by, a face mask, or a resuscitation bag.

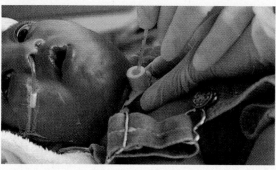

Figure 10-31 *Tracheostomy tube suctioning.*

- Appropriate-size suction catheter
- Sterile container with sterile normal saline

PROCEDURE: *Sterile Gloves*

1. Keep your dominant hand sterile and your nondominant hand clean for the procedure. Use only the dominant hand to manipulate the catheter. With your dominant hand, remove the catheter from the paper sheath, keeping it sterile.

2. Place the distal end of the catheter in a cup of sterile saline to test the suction.

3. With your nondominant hand, remove the humidity source from the child's tracheostomy tube.

4. Oxygenate the child before suctioning, using a resuscitation bag in your nondominant hand. Give several breaths and remove the resuscitation bag.

5. Using your dominant hand, place the suction catheter into the tube, making sure no suction is being applied at this time. Advance the catheter no farther than 0.5 cm below the edge of the tracheostomy tube.

   RATIONALE: *The tracheostomy tube is already fairly far into the trachea. Going deeper may stimulate a vagal response.*

6. Once the catheter is in place, intermittently occlude the suction port and rotate the catheter (Figure 10-31).

7. Remove the catheter and irrigate it in a cup of sterile saline. To prevent the child from becoming hypoxic, do not suction for longer than 5 to 10 seconds.

8. Repeat as necessary, oxygenating between suctionings.

9. Alternately, two people can do the procedure with one applying the resuscitation bag and the other performing suction.

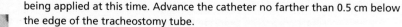

SKILL 10-19 Endotracheal Tube Suctioning

The child with an ET tube is often sedated, so deep suctioning may be required to clear secretions that could obstruct the tube. It must be performed with great care to keep the tube from being dislodged. Hold the tube firmly in place when it is being manipulated, while the ventilator is being disconnected, when the resuscitation bag is being attached and removed, during hyperventilation, and during suctioning.

PREPARATION

1. Use an assistant to help stabilize the ET tube during the procedure.

2. Turn on and set the wall suction to the pressure level ordered by the physician or suggested in the facility's procedure manual. Connect the proximal end of the catheter to the wall suction connection tubing.

3. Turn on the oxygen source attached to the resuscitation bag to inflate the reservoir bag so it is ready for use.

EQUIPMENT AND SUPPLIES

- Appropriate-size suction catheter to fit inside the ET tube (See Table 10-3 on page 97)
- Sterile container with sterile normal saline
- Resuscitator bag
- Oxygen

PROCEDURE: *Sterile Gloves*

1. Keep your dominant hand sterile and your nondominant hand clean for the procedure. Use only the dominant hand to manipulate the catheter.

2. With your dominant hand, remove the catheter from the paper sheath, keeping it sterile. Place the distal end of the catheter in a cup of sterile saline to test the suction pressure.

3. If the child is being ventilated, have an assistant disconnect the ventilator and manually oxygenate the child before suctioning. Give several breaths and then remove the resuscitation bag.

4. Before inserting the catheter, determine how far the suction catheter can be advanced by making a visual comparison of the catheter and the ET tube length.

    RATIONALE: *The visual comparison between the catheter and ET tube length allows for preplanning of how far to advance the catheter to prevent damage to the airway.*

5. With your dominant hand, place the suction catheter into the ET tube, making sure that no suction is being applied at this time. Advance the catheter no farther than 0.5 cm below the edge of the ET tube.

    RATIONALE: *Advancing the catheter beyond this distance has the potential to cause damage to the airway and lungs.*

6. When the catheter is in place, intermittently cover the suction port and rotate the catheter. To prevent the child from becoming hypoxic, do not suction for longer than 5 to 10 seconds.

7. Remove the catheter and irrigate it in a cup of sterile saline. Repeat as necessary, oxygenating the child between suctionings.

Chest Physiotherapy/Postural Drainage

Chest physiotherapy is an airway clearance technique that combines positioning or postural drainage (allowing gravity to help drain secretions into central airways), rhythmic percussion of the chest wall (to help loosen secretions), and coughing and breathing. Chest physiotherapy is used in children who have excessive sputum production or retained bronchial secretions.

These procedures are usually done before the morning meal, and again at bedtime if the child is subject to nighttime mucous retention, plugging of airways, and/or coughing. Chest physiotherapy may be performed more frequently when an infection is present.

Bronchodilators are frequently administered by a handheld nebulizer, intermittent positive pressure breathing (IPPB), or a metered-dose aerosol before drainage is performed.

During postural drainage, two maneuvers can be done to aid in drainage: percussion and vibration (Figure 10-32A and B). Percussion produces chest vibrations that dislodge retained secretions. Vibration is the application of a downward vibrating pressure with the flat part of the palm over the area that is being drained (Figure 10-32C).

> **CLINICAL TIP**
>
> Some children with cystic fibrosis use a vest airway clearance system. The vest provides high-frequency chest wall oscillation that increases airflow velocity to create repetitive coughlike shear forces and to decrease the viscosity of secretions. The vest is used in 30-minute sessions (Goodfellow & Jones, 2002).

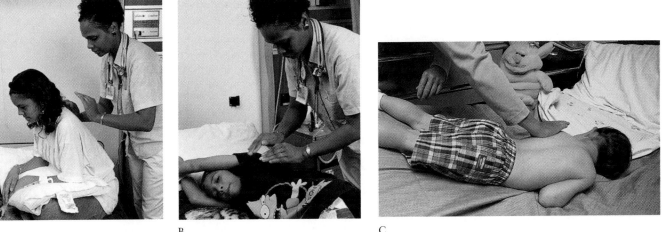

A   B   C

Figure 10-32 *A and B, Postural drainage can be achieved by clapping with a cupped hand on the chest wall over the segment to be drained to create vibrations that are transmitted to the bronchi to dislodge secretions. Various positions are used, depending on the location of the obstruction (see Table 10-4). C, Vibration technique.*

SKILL 10-20 Performing Chest Physiotherapy/Postural Drainage

PREPARATION

1. Ensure that several hours have passed since the child has eaten.
   RATIONALE: *Percussion stimulates coughing spells that can trigger vomiting. Vomiting is less likely if the stomach is empty.*

2. Perform a baseline respiratory assessment. Place the child on a pulse oximeter.
   RATIONALE: *Chest physiotherapy predisposes the child to arterial desaturation. A baseline assessment is used to contrast with the child's responses during the procedure.*

3. Place the child in the position to permit gravity drainage of secretions.

4. Administer the bronchodilator, if ordered, to relax the airway muscles.
   RATIONALE: *When the airway muscles are relaxed, the airway is more dilated so secretions can drain easily.*

EQUIPMENT AND SUPPLIES

- Commercial percussor, round oxygen mask, baby bottle nipple (for infants)
- Vibrator or vibration vest
- Emesis basin or sputum cup
- Pulse oximeter
- Tissues

PROCEDURE: *Percussion*

1. If using the hands to percuss the chest, hold the hands cupped with fingers and thumb together. Keep the wrists loose, elbows partially flexed, and strike the chest alternating the hands. Listen for a hollow sound (see Figures 10-32A and B).

2. Develop a rhythm with the alternate hands and cover the targeted chest area in a circular pattern for 3 to 5 minutes.

3. Avoid tender areas, the breasts of an adolescent girl, and bony prominences such as the clavicles or vertebrae.
   RATIONALE: *Percussion should be focused over intercostal spaces to have the best effect in loosening secretions. Avoiding tender areas will minimize the child's discomfort.*

4. Have the child change position to drain another area of the lungs and percuss that area for 3 to 5 minutes. Continue this process until all areas of the chest have been percussed.

5. The positions used for each patient are based on the location of mucous obstruction (see Table 10-4). In generalized obstructive lung disease, the lower lobes are drained first, followed by the middle lobes and lingula, and the upper lobes are drained last. The various positions used for bronchial drainage in an infant are described in Table 10-5.

6. Encourage the child to take a few deep breaths and to cough after percussion in each location. Have the child expectorate sputum into an emesis basin or cup.
   RATIONALE: *The deep breaths increase the velocity of expired air and help to move the secretions toward the trachea where they can be coughed up.*

7. Monitor the child's cardiorespiratory status.

PROCEDURE: *Vibration*

1. Position one hand flat on the chest over the involved area and the other hand on top of the first. Alternately the hands may be placed side by side on the chest. Keep the arms and shoulders straight (see Figure 10-32C).

2. Tell the child to take a deep breath, inhaling through the nose and exhaling through the mouth.
   RATIONALE: *Vibration is performed only during exhalation.*

3. Vibrate the area by tensing and relaxing your arms for 10 to 15 seconds. Perform these tensing/relaxing actions for 3 to 5 minutes. Move to another area of the chest and repeat the process.

4. Encourage coughing between vibrations and expectoration of sputum into a cup or emesis basin.

TABLE 10-4   Positions Used for Postural Drainage of the Child

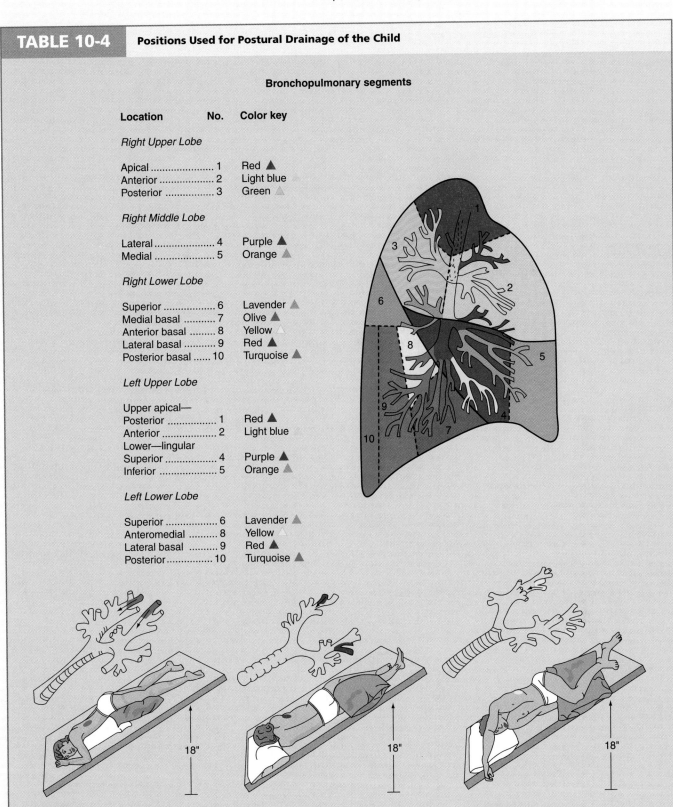

Bronchopulmonary segments

Location	No.	Color key
Right Upper Lobe		
Apical	1	Red ▲
Anterior	2	Light blue
Posterior	3	Green ▲
Right Middle Lobe		
Lateral	4	Purple ▲
Medial	5	Orange ▲
Right Lower Lobe		
Superior	6	Lavender ▲
Medial basal	7	Olive ▲
Anterior basal	8	Yellow △
Lateral basal	9	Red ▲
Posterior basal	10	Turquoise ▲
Left Upper Lobe		
Upper apical—		
Posterior	1	Red ▲
Anterior	2	Light blue
Lower—lingular		
Superior	4	Purple ▲
Inferior	5	Orange ▲
Left Lower Lobe		
Superior	6	Lavender ▲
Anteromedial	8	Yellow △
Lateral basal	9	Red ▲
Posterior	10	Turquoise ▲

Lower Lobes

▲ Posterior Basal Segment (10)

Elevate foot of table or bed 18 in. or 30 degrees. Have child lie prone, head down, with pillow under hips. Upper leg can be flexed over a pillow for support. (Percuss over lower ribs close to spine on each side of chest.)

▲ Lateral Basal Segment (9)

Elevate foot of table or bed 18 in. or 30 degrees. Have child lie prone, then rotate 1/4 turn upward. Upper leg can be flexed over a pillow for support. (Percuss over uppermost portion of lower ribs.)

▲ Anterior Basal Segment (8)

Elevate foot of table or bed 18 in. or 30 degrees. Have child lie on side, head down, pillow under knees. (Percuss over lower ribs just beneath axilla.)

TABLE 10-4   **Positions Used for Postural Drainage of the Child** (continued)

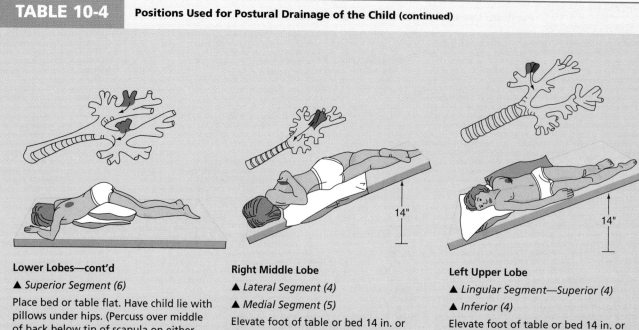

Lower Lobes—cont'd

▲ *Superior Segment (6)*

Place bed or table flat. Have child lie with pillows under hips. (Percuss over middle of back below tip of scapula on either side of spine.)

Right Middle Lobe

▲ *Lateral Segment (4)*

▲ *Medial Segment (5)*

Elevate foot of table or bed 14 in. or about 15 degrees. Have child lie head down on left side and rotate 1/4 turn backward. Pillow may be placed behind child from shoulder to hip. Knees should be flexed. (Percuss over right nipple area.)

Left Upper Lobe

▲ *Lingular Segment—Superior (4)*

▲ *Inferior (4)*

Elevate foot of table or bed 14 in. or about 15 degrees. Have child lie head down on right side and rotate 1/4 turn backward. Pillow may be placed behind child from shoulder to hip. Knees should be flexed. (Percuss over left nipple area.)

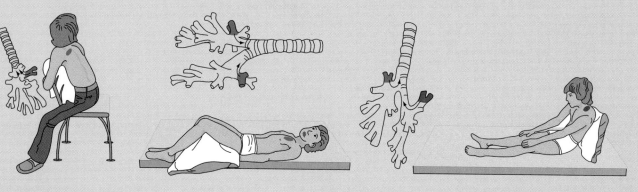

Upper Lobes

▲ *Posterior Segment (3)*

Have child sit up and lean over folded pillow at 30 degree angle. (Percuss over upper back on each side of chest.)

▲ *Anterior Segment (2)*

Place bed or drainage table flat. Have child lie supine with pillow under knees. (Percuss between clavicle and nipple on each side of chest.)

▲ *Apical Segment (1)*

Place bed or drainage table flat. Have child lean back on pillow at 30 degree angle. (Percuss over area between clavicle and top of scapula on each side of chest.)

Modified from material provided by Datalizer Slide Charts, Addison, IL.

TABLE 10-5	Positions to Facilitate Bronchial Drainage in an Infant

Lobes	Percussion/vibration Positions and Locations
Lower lobes	
Posterior basal segment	• Place the infant prone on a pillow on your lap. • Percuss and vibrate the back at the lower ribs.
Lateral basal segment	• Place the infant prone on a pillow on your lap at a 30-degree angle. • Rotate the infant's body slightly so that one side is elevated. • Percuss and vibrate over the lower ribs. • Turn and repeat.
Anterior basal segment	• Extend your legs and keep them slightly flexed (use a chair for support). • Place the infant, supported on a pillow, in a side-lying position (30-degree angle) with the head down. • Percuss and vibrate the area over the ribs under the axilla. • Turn and repeat.
Superior segment	• Place the infant prone on a pillow on your lap • Percuss and vibrate the back.
Upper lobes	
Lateral and medial segments	• Place the infant on your lap in the prone position. • Rotate the infant slightly so that the right side is elevated. • Percuss and vibrate the anterior chest at the nipple. • Turn the infant and repeat.
Posterior segment	• Place the infant on your lap in a sitting position and leaning forward on a pillow at about a 30-degree angle. • Percuss and vibrate both sides of the upper back.
Anterior segment	• Place the infant supine on your lap. • Percuss and vibrate the area between the clavicle and the midchest at the nipple line.
Apical segment	• Place the infant on your lap in a sitting position. Lower the infant to a 30-degree reclining position, using a pillow for support. • Percuss and vibrate the area between the clavicles and the scapulae.

Incentive Spirometry

Incentive spirometry is a method to encourage children to fully expand their lungs to prevent the pooling of secretions that can occur with inactivity.

SKILL 10-21 Using the Incentive Spirometer

PREPARATION

1. Explain the procedure to the child and parents and why it is important to take deep breaths.

2. Identify the incentive spirometer that matches the child's development.

3. If the child has had thoracic or abdominal surgery, show the child and parent how to splint the surgical site to reduce discomfort.

   RATIONALE: *Giving the child some control and a strategy to manage discomfort will lead to increased compliance with the procedure.*

EQUIPMENT AND SUPPLIES

- Incentive spirometer
- Straw and cotton balls or plastic disk
- Pinwheel

PROCEDURE

1. With the incentive spirometer, have the child take a deep breath, close the lips around the tube, and blow forcefully but steadily into the tube to make the ball rise. The blowing should be maintained a few seconds to keep the ball suspended.

2. Repeat the procedure two to three times several times a day. Encourage the child to make the ball rise higher each time until the highest level is reached. After the highest level is reached, encourage the child to lengthen the time the ball is suspended.
   RATIONALE: *The forced, sustained exhalation helps move secretions to the central airway, making it easier to cough them up.*

3. An alternate method is to have the child use a straw to blow cotton balls or a plastic ball across a table. Make the procedure a game.
   RATIONALE: *Children respond to competitions and will work harder to perform the procedure successfully.*

4. Preschool children may respond to blowing a pinwheel. As the pinwheel's spinning slows, have the child take another deep breath and blow again. Encourage the child to stretch the expiration to make the pinwheel spin longer. When the child is able to blow more forcefully, slowly move the pinwheel further away.

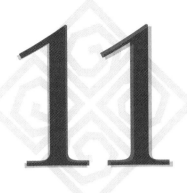

11

Nutrition

Chapter Outline

Gastric Tubes

Gastric tubes are used in infants and children to provide a means of alimentation and to decompress or empty the stomach. The size of the nasogastric or orogastric tube is determined by the age, size, and weight of the child.

Orogastric Tubes

Orogastric tubes are used in newborns and young infants who are obligate nose breathers, and in older children who are unconscious, unresponsive, or intubated.

SKILL 11-1 Inserting and Removing an Orogastric Tube

PREPARATION

1. Place the child supine with the head of the bed elevated, unless contraindicated.

2. Use the tube to measure the distance from the mouth to the tragus of the ear and then to the xiphoid process to determine the distance to the stomach. (Alternatively, use a point midway between the xiphoid and the umbilicus.) Mark the tube with tape.

EQUIPMENT AND SUPPLIES

- Appropriate-size orogastric tube
- Suction catheter
- Water-soluble lubricant
- Stethoscope
- 20-mL syringe to check tube placement

PROCEDURE: *Clean Gloves*

Insertion

1. Have suction at hand. Apply a water-soluble lubricant to the tube.

2. Position the child with the neck slightly hyperextended. Open the child's mouth and insert the tube toward the back of the throat. Continue advancing the tube slowly until you reach the mark.
   RATIONALE: *This position facilitates passage of the tube by opening the neck and mouth.*

3. Check the tube for placement by aspirating the stomach contents and checking the pH; a pH of 3 or below indicates stomach placement. An alternate method of checking placement is to auscultate over the abdomen while a small amount of air (5 mL or up to 10 mL for an older child) is injected through the tube into the stomach. Sometimes an x-ray is used to verify correct placement. Assess the child's respiratory status and color. A change in either may indicate that the tube is located in the trachea rather than in the esophagus.

4. Once you are assured that the tube is in place, tape it securely to one side of the child's mouth. Place two pieces of tape in a V pattern around the tube at the lip. If necessary, use a third piece of tape over the other two. Clamp the end of the tube if it is not being used for feeding or suctioning.
   RATIONALE: *Measures must be taken to maintain the tube in correct position so that it does not become dislodged.*

Removal

1. Have suction available.
   RATIONALE: *If the child vomits it may be necessary to remove secretions.*

2. Instill approximately 10 to 20 mL of air into the tube to remove any secretions.

3. Untape the tube, pinch or fold it to prevent fluid leakage, and gently withdraw it.

Nasogastric Tubes

Nasogastric tubes are used more frequently than orogastric tubes. They are inserted to provide alimentation, to decompress the stomach, or to empty the stomach of its contents in preparation for surgery or lavage.

SKILL 11-2 Inserting and Removing a Nasogastric Tube

PREPARATION

1. Tell the preschool-age child what will happen in very simple terms. Give the school-age child and adolescent a rationale for the procedure. Because tube placement is uncomfortable, allow the child to express his or her feelings and seek the support of family members.

2. Place the child supine, with the head of the bed elevated to the high-Fowler's position, if possible. Restrain younger children because they will fight against the insertion of the tube. An assistant can hold the child's body and arms with the body, or the child can be put in a modified mummy restraint. The child's head must be held in the midline position.

3. Use the tube to measure the distance from the tip of the nose to the tragus of the ear and then to the xiphoid process to determine the distance to the stomach (Figure 11-1). (Alternatively, use a point midway between the xiphoid and the umbilicus.) Mark the tube with tape.

EQUIPMENT AND SUPPLIES

- Appropriate-size nasogastric tube
- Suction catheter
- Water-soluble lubricant
- Stethoscope
- 20-mL syringe to check tube placement

PROCEDURE: *Clean Gloves*

Insertion

1. Have suction at hand. Apply water-soluble lubricant to the distal end of the tube.

2. With the child's neck slightly hyperextended, insert the tube into the child's naris, gently advancing it straight back along the floor of the nasal passages. If resistance is felt at the curve of the nasopharynx, use slight pressure or rotate the tube to continue advancing it.

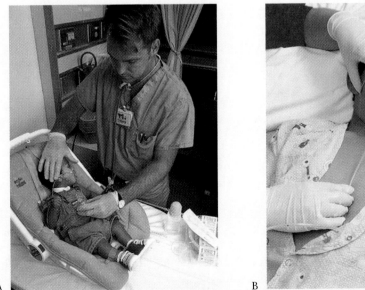

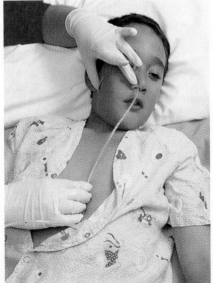

Figure 11-1 *Measuring for nasogastric tube placement in A, infant, and B, child. (A similar technique is used in measuring for orogastric tube insertion. See the previous discussion.)*

A   B

3. If the child gags when the tube reaches beyond the oropharynx, flex the child's neck. If the child can take fluids by mouth, have him or her sip water through a straw and swallow it to ease the passage of the tube over the glottis. If the child is not allowed anything by mouth, have him or her swallow.

      RATIONALE: *Gagging is most common as the tube passes just beyond the back of the throat. Swallowing can decrease the gag reflex until the tube is advanced slightly beyond this point.*

4. After the gag reflex is suppressed, continue advancing the tube slowly until you reach the mark.

5. Check the tube for placement by aspirating the stomach contents and checking the pH; a pH of 3 or under indicates placement in the stomach. An alternate method of checking placement is to auscultate over the abdomen while a small amount of air (5 mL or up to 10 mL for older children) is injected through the tube into the stomach (Figure 11-2). Sometimes an x-ray is used to verify correct placement. Assess the child's respiratory status and color. A change in either may indicate that the tube is located in the trachea rather than in the esophagus.

6. Once you are assured that the tube is in place, tape it securely by placing two pieces of tape in a V pattern around the tube and attaching it to the nose or cheek (Figure 11-3). If necessary, use a second piece of tape over the first.

Removal

1. Have suction available.

2. Place the child in a Fowler's position.

3. Instill approximately 10 to 15 mL of air into the tube to remove any secretions.

4. Unfasten the tape, ask the child to hold his or her breath, pinch the tube, and gently pull it out.

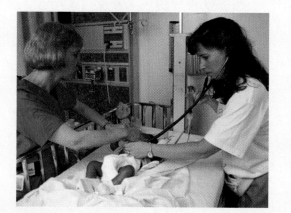

Figure 11-2 *Checking for nasogastric tube placement.*

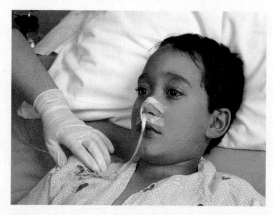

Figure 11-3 *Nasogastric tube taped securely in place.*

Gastrostomy Tubes

Gastrostomy tubes are surgically placed in the stomach and are used primarily for gavage feeding. The tube should remain clamped when it is not being used for feeding or decompression.

    Observe the site for skin breakdown. Keep the area clean and dry. Place a clean, dry dressing over the site at every shift. A 2 × 2 or 4 × 4 inch gauze pad can be used. A diagonal cut is made halfway into the square and placed around the tube with tape used at the edges to secure it.

    Keep the tube as immobile as possible to prevent unintentional removal or displacement. Tube placement can be checked by aspirating a small amount of gastric contents before each feeding.

    The gastrostomy feeding button is a flexible silicone device that is often used for children who require long-term enteral feedings.

Gavage/Tube Feeding

Infants and children require gavage or tube feeding to counteract absorption disorders, to provide supplemental feedings, and to conserve calories for growth. Feedings can be either continuous or bolus. They can be administered by gravity (Figure 11-4) or by pump (Figures 11-5A and B). A pump is preferred because it permits good regulation of the rate and volume of the feeding.

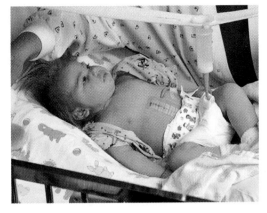

Figure 11-4 *Gavage feeding by gravity.*

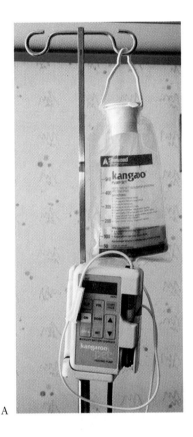

A

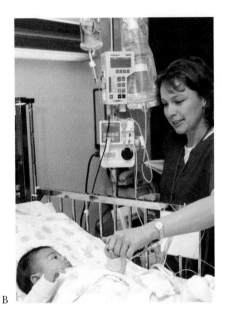

B

Figure 11-5 *A, Feeding pump. B, The pump helps regulate the rate and volume of feeding.*

SKILL 11-3 Administering a Gavage/Tube Feeding

PREPARATION

1. If the feeding is to be given by gravity, an IV pole may be used. If the feeding is to be given by pump, gather the necessary bag and tubing. Prime the appropriate tubing, keeping the distal end covered.

   RATIONALE: *The tubing is primed to eliminate air. If air is infused into the gastrointestinal tract, discomfort can occur.*

2. If possible, place the child in a semi-Fowler's position. If not, a prone or side-lying position is preferred to the supine position.

   RATIONALE: *These positions decrease the risk of aspiration.*

EQUIPMENT AND SUPPLIES

- Formula at room temperature (to prevent cramping)
- Water for irrigation of the tube
- Stethoscope
- 20-mL syringe to check tube placement

PROCEDURE: *Clean Gloves*

1. Check the placement of the tube before each feeding by aspirating the stomach contents or auscultating over the abdomen while a small amount of air (5 mL or 10 mL in older children) is injected through the tube into the stomach.

2. Assess the child's respiratory status and color.
   RATIONALE: *Changes in either may indicate that the nasogastric or orogastric tube is located in the trachea instead of in the esophagus.*

3. Once you are assured that the tube is in place, check gastric residuals and proceed with the steps necessary for the feeding.

Bolus Feeding

1. Aspirate the stomach contents to check the amount of residual. If the residual is less than half of the previous feeding, return the aspirated contents to the stomach. If the residual is greater, notify the physician.
   RATIONALE: *Large residual indicates that the child is not absorbing the feeding. Type or amount may need adjustment.*

2. Attach the primed tubing from either the pump or the gravity set to the gastrostomy tube. Start the flow slowly while checking the patency of the tube. Set the rate and volume according to the physician's orders.

3. When the feeding has been completed, assess the child's condition. Clamp and disconnect the tubing. Flush the tubing with a small amount of water to clean it.

4. When families will carry out tube feedings at home, be sure that they understand the procedure and what to do for any problems (see Table 11-1).

TABLE 11-1	Home Care Instructions for the Child Requiring Gastrostomy Tube Feedings and Care

Equipment

Prepared, prescribed feeding
Enteral feeding pump
Long-nosed syringe

Procedure

1. Wash hands.
2. Warm prescribed formula to room temperature.
3. Pour formula to run through the feeding bag.
4. Allow formula to run through the tubing to remove air. Close clamp.
5. Attach syringe to the end of the gastrostomy tube. Unclamp the gastrostomy tube.
6. Pull plunger back until resistance is felt. Check amount of formula in syringe. If more than half of the prescribed amount is withdrawn, refer to the section on problem solving (below). If less than the prescribed amount is withdrawn, push the formula gently back through the syringe.
7. Instill water through the tube.
8. Attach the feeding bag to the gastrostomy tube. Infuse at the prescribed rate.
9. Burp or bubble the infant throughout the feeding.
10. After feeding, flush the gastrostomy tube with water and clamp the tube.
11. Position the infant prone or side lying for 30–60 min after feedings.

Psychosocial Needs

Hold and rock the infant or child during feedings.
Give a pacifier to an infant or a bottle or cup to a child to meet developmental needs.

TABLE 11-1	Home Care Instructions for the Child Requiring Gastrostomy Tube Feedings and Care (continued)

Medication Administration

Use liquid medication when possible.

Crush only uncoated tablets.

Crush tablets to a fine powder and mix with water or juice.

Flush tubing before and after medication administration.

Stoma Care

Wash the area around the stoma twice a day with soap and water.

Use half-strength hydrogen peroxide to remove any crusting.

Look for signs of infection such as redness, swelling, and discharge.

Notify the physician if any signs of infection or leakage are present.

Problem Solving

Problem	Cause	Action
Formula will not flow	Blocked tube (clamping, foreign material) Viscous formula	Check clamp. Reposition. Pull back on syringe. Instill water. Milk tube. Notify physician.
	Pump malfunction	Check plug. Call company. Give feeding by gravity.
Large volume of undigested formula removed before feeding	Delayed absorption	Reinfuse remaining formula. If more than half of feeding, subtract from the next feeding. Do not discard the residual.
	Constipation	Check for last bowel movement. Notify primary care provider.
Constipation	Decreased free fluids	Give water and juice between feedings as tolerated. Report bowel problems or hard stools to primary care provider.
Diarrhea	Hyperosmolar formula Rapid rate of flow Cold formula	Dilute formula. Feed at a slower rate. Warm formula to room temperature before feeding.
	Bacterial contamination	Treat with antibiotics.
Dislodged tube	Inadequate stabilization	Bring child for emergency care
Skin irritation	Formula leakage	Skin care; barrier if needed

Note: From Borkowski, S. (1998). Pediatric stomas, tubes, and appliances. *Pediatric Clinics of North America, 45,* 1419–1435; Young, C., & White, S. (1992). Preparing patients for tube feeding at home. *American Journal of Nursery, 92,* 46–53.

Continuous Feeding

1. The procedure for continuous feeding is very similar to that for bolus feeding; however, the formula should hang no longer than 4 hours.

    RATIONALE: *Microorganisms can grow in warm formula, so it must be changed if left out for several hours.*

2. When the feeding bag is hung, label it with the time and date.

3. Change the feeding set once per shift or every 8 hours.

4. Assess the child's condition and monitor respiratory status during the feeding.

Gastric Suctioning

Both orogastric and nasogastric tubes can be connected to a suctioning device (Figure 11-6) to provide either continuous or intermittent suction.

Figure 11-6 *Nasogastric tube attached to a suctioning device.*

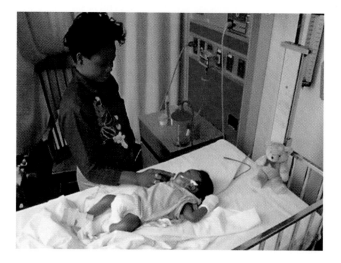

SKILL 11-4 Performing Gastric Suctioning

PREPARATION: *Clean Gloves*

1. Before making the connection, don gloves.
2. Check the suction equipment.
3. Check the tube for proper position by aspirating the stomach contents or auscultating over the abdomen while a small amount of air (5 mL or 10 mL in older children) is injected through the tube into the stomach.
4. Assess the child's respiratory status and color. Changes in either may indicate that the tube is located in the trachea instead of in the esophagus.

EQUIPMENT AND SUPPLIES

- Suctioning equipment
- Stethescope
- 10-mL syringe for air insertion

PROCEDURE

1. Attach the suction to the orogastric or nasogastric tube at its distal end. Tape the connection site.
2. Turn the suction to the setting ordered by the physician. Observe the color, amount, and character of the contents suctioned.
3. Record the child's response (vital signs, complaints of abdominal discomfort).
4. Monitor the child's condition frequently and label the level of the contents collected.
   RATIONALE: *Contents can indicate difficulty absorbing nutrients or suggest problems with digestive processes. In the case of suction following poisoning, contents can indicate amount of poisonous substance that has been successfully removed.*

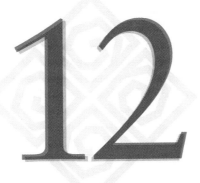

12

Elimination

Chapter Outline

Urinary Catheterization

Urinary catheterization is performed to obtain sterile urine for diagnostic purposes, to measure the amount of urine in the bladder accurately, to empty the bladder, or to relieve bladder distention. In the hospital setting it is performed as a sterile procedure. For children outside the hospital who need intermittent catheterization, it is done as a clean procedure.

SKILL 12-1 Performing a Urinary Catheterization

PREPARATION

1. Check the physician's orders to determine if intermittent or indwelling catheterization is planned.

2. Determine the size of the catheter based on the child's size, age, and weight.

3. Explain the procedure to the child and parent and why it is necessary.

4. Have an assistant hold the child in position for the procedure. If the parents wish to stay with the child, have them stand at the child's head and try to distract the child.

5. Place absorbent pads under the child's perineum.

6. Open the tray, maintaining the sterile field. Open the lubricant and squeeze it onto the sterile field. Pour the antiseptic over the cotton swabs or balls.

7. Put on sterile gloves. Lubricate the tip of the catheter and place the distal end in the tray.

EQUIPMENT AND SUPPLIES

- Urinary catheter—size appropriate for the child's age, and one a size smaller
- Sterile urinary catheterization tray (containing drapes, sterile gloves, antiseptic solution, cotton swabs or balls, forceps, lubricant, and a container for urine)
- A container for soiled cotton balls
- Syringe filled with normal saline
- Tape
- Drainage collection apparatus
- Absorbent pads

PROCEDURE

Female

1. Clean the perineum. Spread the labia apart with the nondominant hand. Pick up the antiseptic-soaked cotton balls with forceps using the dominant hand. Clean the meatus, using one ball for each wipe, in a front-to-back direction along each side of the labia minora, then along the sides of the urinary meatus, and finally straight down over the urethral opening. Discard each cotton ball away from the sterile field.
   RATIONALE: *Wipe in the direction from the urinary meatus toward the anus to avoid contaminating the urinary meatus with fecal bacteria.*

2. Pick up the lubricated catheter tip with the dominant hand, keeping the distal end in the specimen container.
   RATIONALE: *The dominant hand remains sterile and should only handle the catheter. Placing the distal end in a specimen container prevents contamination of the sterile field when urine flows.*

3. Gently insert the tip into the meatus (approximately 5 to 8 cm [2 to 3 in] in the child) until there is a free flow of urine, and then 2.5 cm (1 in) further. If resistance is felt, do not force the catheter. Try again with another sterile catheter, preferably one size smaller.
   RATIONALE: *A catheter should not be used a second time to prevent potential infection in the child.*

CLINICAL TIP

Recommended Urinary Catheter Sizes

Infant: 4–5 French

Toddler and preschooler: 6 French

School-age child: 6–10 French

Adolescent: 8–12 French

4. When the catheter is in place, collect the urine specimen and drain the bladder while holding the distal end of the catheter with the nondominant hand. Handle the urine specimen as described in Chapter 6. Remove the tube.

5. For an indwelling catheter, attach tubing to the drainage apparatus. Tape the tubing to the leg to avoid pulling.

6. Use the syringe to inflate the balloon on the catheter to the recommended amount of normal saline.

7. Make sure the tubing has no kinks. Hang the drainage apparatus on the bed frame.

PROCEDURE

Male

1. Clean the perineum. With the nondominant hand, hold the penis behind the glans and spread the meatus with the thumb and forefinger. Retract the foreskin if the child is uncircumcised.

2. Use the dominant hand to pick up the forceps and antiseptic-soaked cotton balls. Clean the tissue surrounding the meatus using one cotton ball for each wipe in an outward circular motion. Discard each cotton ball away from the sterile field.

3. Pick up the lubricated catheter tip with the dominant hand, and place the distal end in a specimen container. Lift the penis, exerting slight traction until it is perpendicular to the body. Insert the catheter steadily into the meatus until urine begins to flow, and then about 2.5 cm (1 in) further (up to a total of 10 to 12 cm [5 to 6 in] maximum).
   RATIONALE: *The catheter is inserted an extra inch into the bladder to ensure proper placement for drainage when an indwelling catheter is planned.*

4. If resistance to the catheter is felt, have the child blow out to relax the perineal muscles. Do not force the catheter. Another catheter, one size smaller, may be used if relaxation efforts are not successful.

5. Once the catheter is in place, lower the penis and collect the urine specimen while holding the distal end of the catheter with the nondominant hand. Handle the urine specimen as described in Chapter 6. Remove the tube.

6. For an indwelling catheter, attach tubing to the drainage apparatus. Tape the tubing to the leg to avoid pulling.

7. Use the syringe to inflate the balloon on the catheter to the recommended amount of normal saline.

8. Make sure the tubing has no kinks. Hang the drainage apparatus on the bed frame.

SKILL 12-2 Double Diapering With a Stent in Place

A double diapering technique is used to protect the stent (small tube that drains urine) following repair of hypospadius or epispadius.

PROCEDURE

1. Open two diapers on top of each other and place under the infant's perineum.

2. Hold the stent to the side and place the first diaper over the perineum. Position the stent to drain into the second diaper. Fold the second diaper into place (Figure 12-1).
   RATIONALE: *This process prevents contamination of the stent with feces. Urinary output and urine color can be assessed post surgery.*

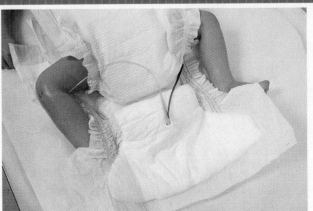

Figure 12-1 *A double diapering technique protects the urinary stent after surgery for hypospadias or epispadias repair. The inner diaper collects stool; the outer diaper, urine.*

Ostomy Care

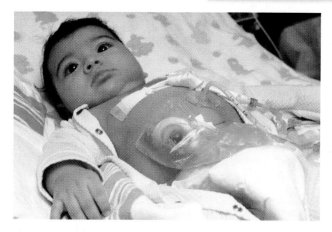

Figure 12-2 *This infant has several gastrointestinal problems and requires ostomies both for gastric feedings and for drainage of fecal material. The care of the skin is challenging and important for this infant to prevent infection and provide adequate nutrition.*

Ostomies are performed when an infant or child requires fecal or urinary diversion (Figure 12-2). Infants and children may require an ostomy for several reasons, including necrotizing enterocolitis, Hirschsprung's disease, imperforate anus, prune-belly syndrome, inflammatory bowel syndrome, spina bifida, tumor, and trauma. An ileostomy, colostomy, or urinary diversion is performed depending on the disorder and its location.

An adhesive appliance is usually applied just after surgery to measure drainage. If a dressing is applied instead of an adhesive appliance, the drainage can be measured by weighing the dressing both before and after saturation. For each 1-g increase in weight of the dressing, approximately 1 mL of fluid has drained into it.

In children and infants, ostomies pose special problems because of the fragility of the skin. Care must be taken to prevent skin breakdown at the site.

SKILL 12-3 Changing the Dressing for an Infant With an Ostomy

CLINICAL TIP

Avoid adhesive enhancers on the skin of newborns and prematures. Their skin is so thin that removal of the appliance can strip off the skin. Remember that adhesive contains latex and it should not be used in those who are latex sensitive or allergic.

PREPARATION

1. Observe drainage on the dressing carefully so it can be described in documentation.

EQUIPMENT AND SUPPLIES

- Gauze
- Tape or other supplies to hold gauze in place

PROCEDURE: *Clean Gloves*

1. After each bowel movement, don gloves, change the dressing, clean and dry the skin, and apply a nonporous substance.

   RATIONALE: *Fecal matter and intestinal fluids can cause skin breakdown. Measures must be taken to prevent this complication.*

2. Observe the stoma for complications.

   RATIONALE: *Common complications in children include prolapse, retraction, stenosis, and skin breakdown.*

3. To absorb drainage, place gauze with slits cut to fit around the stoma. Use tape to hold the gauze in place. Alternatively, Montgomery straps, an Ace wrap, or a diaper can be used to hold the gauze in place.

   RATIONALE: *Tape sometimes irritates the fragile skin of infants and other methods could be used to protect the skin.*

Note: Once the stoma has healed and the infant is large enough to wear a pouch, an appliance with a Stomahesive wafer will be used.

SKILL 12-4 Changing an Ostomy Pouch for an Infant or Child

PREPARATION

1. Describe the procedure to the child if it has not been performed before.

2. Ask parents and child about procedures used at home if the child has had the ostomy for some time.

EQUIPMENT AND SUPPLIES

- Pouch and clamp
- Stomahesive or other pectin wafer
- Water and washcloth or gauze
- Towel or gauze
- Pads for bed
- Bag for discarding used materials

PROCEDURE: *Clean Gloves*

1. Don gloves.

2. Place a pad on bed to protect it from drainage.

3. Empty the pouch when one-third to one-half full. Remove the pouch, and place it in a sealable plastic bag for disposal.

4. Children will commonly have Stomahesive around the stoma.
   RATIONALE: *Stomahesive is a wafer of protective material to which a pouch can be attached or removed, thus protecting the integrity of the skin. Most wafers require changing only once a week.*

5. Wash the skin and the stoma gently with water and soap without oil. Note any skin breakdown or signs of infection. Dry the area.

6. Prepare the new pouch.

7. Measure the Stomahesive or wafer so that it fits exactly around the stoma. Place it securely on the dried skin. Press the pouch firmly against the Stomahesive to form a tight seal. Be careful to avoid making any wrinkles. Close the opening of the pouch with the appropriate clamp.
   RATIONALE: *Measures are taken to prevent fecal matter from leaking onto skin surface where it could cause breakdown. During the immediate postoperative period, the size of the stoma can change, so careful measurement of the wafer to avoid skin damage by fecal material is needed.*

Enemas

The three important considerations when giving an enema to an infant or a child are the type of fluid, the amount of fluid, and the appropriate distance to insert the tube into the rectum (see Table 12-1).

Generally, an isotonic fluid such as normal saline is used for children; however, a commercial hypertonic product, such as a pediatric Fleet enema, is sometimes used.

TABLE 12-1	Guidelines for Enema Administration to Children	

Age	Volume (mL)	Distance for Inserting Tube
Infant	40–100	2.5 cm (1 in)
Toddler	100–200	5.0 cm (2 in)
Preschooler	200–300	5.0 cm (2 in)
School-age child	300–500	7.5 cm (3 in)
Adolescent	500–700	10.0 cm (4 in)

SKILL 12-5 Administering an Enema

PREPARATION

1. Explain the procedure to the child. Assure the child that a bedpan will be kept at bedside.

2. If the child is toilet trained, place him or her in a bed near a bathroom before giving the enema.

3. Ensure privacy.

EQUIPMENT AND SUPPLIES

- Ordered solution (in container with attached tip) *or* enema bag and rectal tube (size 14 to 18 French for child; 12 French for infant)
- Solution container
- Ordered fluid
- Water-soluble lubricant
- Pads for bed

PROCEDURE: *Clean Gloves*

1. Don gloves.

2. Place absorbent pads on the bed. Position the child on his or her left side, with the knees drawn up to the chest or right leg flexed over the left leg. You may need an assistant to hold the child in position.
   RATIONALE: *When the child is on the left side, entry of the fluid into the colon is facilitated.*

3. If a rectal tube is being used, attach the solution container, add the fluid, and purge the tubing and tube. Lubricate the tip. If a Fleet enema is used, prelubricate the tip.

4. Gently insert the tip to the recommended distance. Allow the fluid to run in slowly, for at least 10 to 15 minutes. If the child complains of cramping, stop the infusion to allow the child to rest, then continue.

5. Infants and children may not be able to retain the fluid. Holding the buttocks together might help.

6. When the child is ready or when it is time to expel the contents of the enema, place the bedpan on the bed or escort the child to the bathroom. Provide privacy as requested. Assess for dizziness or weakness before leaving.

7. Clean the perineum. The child or parent may choose to perform this step.

8. Help the child resume a position of comfort.

9. Assess the return for amount and character.

Musculoskeletal Care

Chapter Outline

Casts

Crutches

Braces

Traction

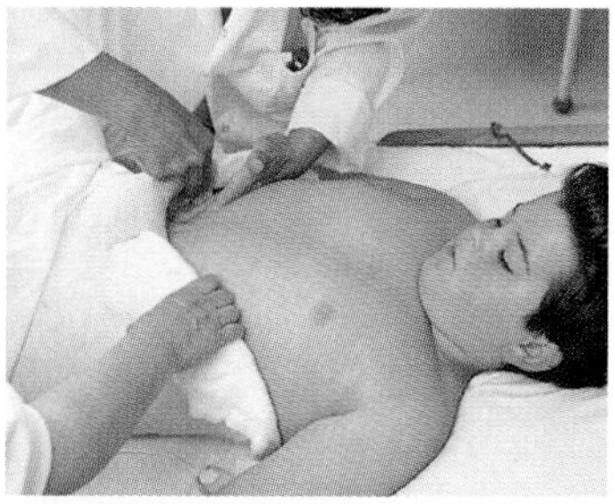

Figure 13-1 *Nurses check the edges of the fresh cast for dryness and roughness.*

Casts

Children often have casts applied after surgery or to treat fractures. They may have white plaster casts that are generally heavy and sturdy. Alternatively, fiberglass casts are lighter, come in various colors, but generally do not last as long. Nurses may assist with cast application, and are involved in immediate cast care after application. They commonly instruct the child and family on maintenance of the cast at home. The following procedure describes the nurse's role in care after cast application. See Chapter 21 of *Pediatric Nursing: Caring for Children, Third Edition,* for further information about management of musculoskeletal treatments (Figure 13-1).

SKILL 13-1 Providing Cast Care

PREPARATION

1. Consult the child's chart for a description of the injury or surgery.

EQUIPMENT AND SUPPLIES

- Cast material (if assisting in application)
- Large basin with water (if assisting in application)
- Pillows with waterproof covering
- Absorbent pads and protectors

PROCEDURE: *Clean Gloves*

1. Elevate a wet cast on pillows covered in plastic.
   RATIONALE: *Elevation decreases edema under the cast which can restrict circulation.*

2. Use the palm of the hands when lifting a wet or damp cast.
   RATIONALE: *Fingertips can indent plaster and create pressure areas.*

3. Circle and note date and time of any drainage on the cast.
   RATIONALE: *Some drainage is common after surgery. Monitoring its presence provides clues to the amount and type of fluid lost.*

4. Assess circulation and neurological status every 15 minutes immediately after surgery or cast placement and then progress to every 30 minutes, 60 minutes, and 2 hours. Report abnormal findings or changes in condition. Include the following observations on the involved extremities:
   - Distal pulses
   - Color
   - Warmth
   - Capillary refill
   - Edema
   - Movement
   - Pain, tingling
   - Sensation

   RATIONALE: *Circulation and nerves under the cast can be injured if it is too tight.*

5. Check the edges of the cast for roughness or crumbling. Pull the inner stockinette over the edge of the cast and tape once the cast has dried.
   RATIONALE: *These actions can prevent discomfort and skin breakdown.*

6. Keep the cast clean and dry. Cover it with a plastic bag during bathing or toileting.
7. Avoid use of lotions and powders under the cast.
   RATIONALE: *These products can cause skin irritation.*

8. Keep shirts or other clothing over the top edges of casts on young children.
   RATIONALE: *This action helps to prevent the child from placing objects down into the cast which can result in areas of discomfort or skin damage.*

NURSING ALERT

Neurovascular impairment under a cast is an emergency. If assessments indicate impaired circulation or neurological status, notify the physician immediately. Have a cast cutter at the bedside so the cast can quickly be removed if needed and the pressure relieved.

9. Instruct the family about care of the cast at home and when to return for checks and removal of the cast (see Table 13-1).

TABLE 13-1	Home Care Instructions for the Care of the Child with a Cast

Skin Care

- Check the skin around the cast edges for irritation, rubbing, or blistering. The skin should be clean and dry.
- You may cleanse the skin just under the cast edges and between the toes or fingers with a cotton-tipped applicator and rubbing alcohol. Avoid using lotions, oils, and powders near the cast as they may cause caking.
- Avoid poking sharp objects down inside the cast as this may result in sores.

Cast Care

- Keep the cast dry. Protect plaster with a cast shoe, thick sock, or sling.
- Allow a new, wet cast to air-dry for 24 hours.
- You may begin walking on a leg cast only if your physician has given you permission to do so.

Be Alert for Possible Complications

- Toes or fingers should be pink, not blue or white.
- Skin should be warm and the tips of the toes should blanch when pinched.
- Raise the casted arm or leg above heart level and rest it on pillows to prevent or reduce any swelling.

Notify Your Health Care Provider If Any of the Following Occur

- Unusual odor beneath the cast
- Tingling
- Burning or numbness in the casted arm or leg
- Drainage through the cast
- Swelling or inability to move the fingers or toes
- Slippage of the cast
- Cast cracked, soft, or loose
- Sudden unexplained fever
- Unusual fussiness or irritability in an infant or child
- Fingers or toes that are blue or white
- Pain that is not relieved by any comfort measures (i.e., repositioning or pain medication)

Note: Courtesy of Shriners Hospital for Children, Spokane, WA. Adapted.

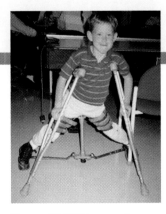

Figure 13-2 *This young boy uses crutches to walk while in the Toronto brace for treatment of Perthes disease.*

Crutches

Children may need crutches temporarily after surgery or injury of an extremity, or permanently to assist in ambulation. Crutches are generally supported under the axilla, or for long-term use, may be supported by an attachment fitting over the forearm (Canadian crutches). Nurses assist children to learn to walk safely with crutches, ensure that children using crutches over time are evaluated as needed for correct fit, and monitor the skin that receives pressure from the crutches (Figure 13-2).

SKILL 13-2 Setting Crutch Height

PROCEDURE

- While standing, have the child's elbows slightly and comfortably flexed.
- Place the tip of the crutches about 3 to 6 inches from upper, outer border of the toes on each foot.
- The upper pad on the crutches should now be lightly placed in the child's axilla.

   RATIONALE: *Crutches that are too high can put pressure on the brachial plexus, causing pain and injury. Crutches that are too low require that the child bend over to walk, and thus can injure or cause discomfort of the back and neck.*

Braces

Braces are used to treat conditions temporarily (such as for scoliosis in a teenager), or may be used on a long-term basis (such as a child with cerebral palsy who needs leg braces for ambulation). The nurse helps the child accommodate to new braces and then periodically evaluates the fit of the braces and the condition of the skin. Brace wear is usually part of the home and community nursing role. See Table 13-2 for guidelines to teach families about brace wear.

TABLE 13-2	Guidelines for Brace Wear

- Braces should be as comfortable as possible and the child should have adequate mobility while wearing the brace.
- Begin wearing the brace for periods of 1–2 hours and then progress to 2–4 hours.
- Check the skin every 1–2 hours initially, then lengthening to every 4 hours once skin has been clear for several days. If redness is apparent, leave the brace off and allow the skin to clear. If breakdown has occurred, the brace cannot be replaced until healing is complete.
- Always have the child wear a clean white sock, T-shirt, or other thin white liner beneath the brace. Be sure the liner is wrinkle-free under the brace. Avoid using powders or lotions that can cause skin to break down. Toughen any sensitive areas using alcohol wipes.
- Reapply the brace when the skin returns to its normal color.
- Return to the physicion or orthotic specialist if discomfort or red areas persist or if the brace needs adjustment or repair or is outgrown.
- Check the brace daily for rough edges.

Traction

Various types of traction are used to provide force on bones and muscles. Skin or external traction is sometimes used, while skeletal or internal traction involves surgery to place pins into bones which are then attached to traction apparatus. The nurse sets up the type of traction ordered and maintains it while monitoring the patient for response and condition. See Chapter 21 in *Pediatric Nursing: Caring for Children, Third Edition,* for types of traction.

SKILL 13-3 Applying Traction

PREPARATION

1. Explain to the child and family the type of traction and what it will involve.

2. Gather equipment needed and review proper setup.

3. Check the weights to be certain they are the same as those ordered by the physician.

EQUIPMENT AND SUPPLIES

- Poles, pulleys, rope, weight, pads
- Elastic wrap for external traction

PROCEDURE

1. Set up prescribed type of traction with proper weights.

2. Apply traction as ordered to particular extremity.

3. Perform assessments every 30 minutes initially, and then advance to 1 to 2 hours when stable. Areas to include are as follows:

   - Proper position of traction
   - Neurovascular status of extremity (see previous discussion on cast care)
   - Skin condition under and around traction application
   - Skin on prominences exposed to surface of bed
   - Vital signs
   - Pain and psychological status

   RATIONALE: *Traction can lead to skin breakdown or neurovascular impairment. Infections can result, especially with internal traction. Regular assessments help to identify problems early. Children may be pulled out of correct alignment by traction and movement in bed and may require frequent repositioning.*

4. Perform sterile pin care as ordered or according to agency policy for the child with internal traction.

   RATIONALE: *Pin care helps to keep the insertion sites clean and minimizes the chance of infection.*

5. Provide teaching and evaluation of technique if the family will maintain traction at home (Figure 13-3).

HOME CARE CONSIDERATIONS

Children are increasingly being treated with traction at home. Be certain that the family understands how to set up and maintain the traction. Teach the observations to be made on the extremity involved. Siblings may change the weights or ropes so close supervision may be needed by parents in some families. A home visit soon after traction begins is often made to evaluate the family's understanding and ability to carry out the regimen.

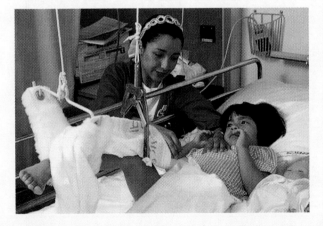

Figure 13-3 *The child in traction needs close monitoring for alignment and proper traction application. Parents can often provide distraction and activities to help children pass the time during their immobility.*

Appendix A: Physical Growth Charts

Physical growth percentiles for length and weight—boys: birth to 36 months.
From CDC, 2001.
www.cdc.gov/growthcharts

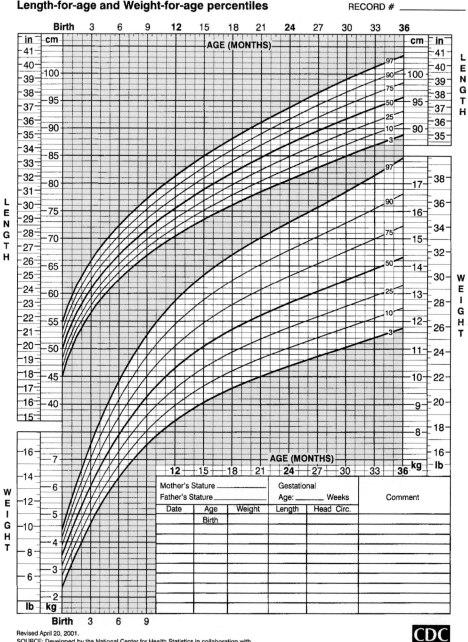

Birth to 36 months: Boys
Length-for-age and Weight-for-age percentiles

NAME _____

RECORD # _____

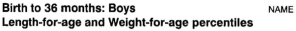

Revised April 20, 2001.
SOURCE: Developed by the National Center for Health Statistics in collaboration with
the National Center for Chronic Disease Prevention and Health Promotion (2000).
http://www.cdc.gov/growthcharts

CDC

Birth to 36 months: Boys
Head circumference-for-age and
Weight-for-length percentiles

NAME _____

RECORD # _____

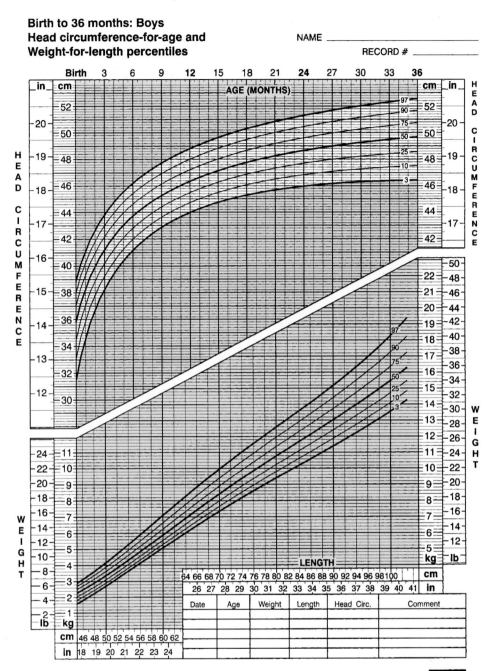

SOURCE: Developed by the National Center for Health Statistics in collaboration with
the National Center for Chronic Disease Prevention and Health Promotion (2000).
http://www.cdc.gov/growthcharts

FIGURE A-2 ◆

Physical growth percentiles for
head circumference, weight for
length—boys: birth to 36 months.
From CDC, 2001.
www.cdc.gov/growthcharts

FIGURE A-3 ◆

Physical growth percentiles for
length and weight—girls: birth to
36 months.
From CDC, 2001.
www.cdc.gov/growthcharts

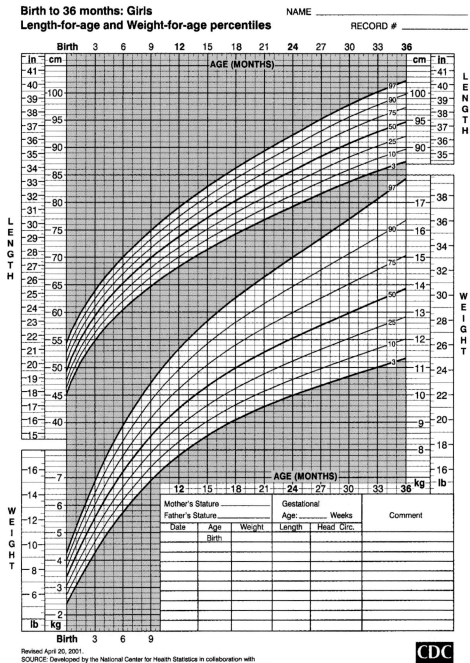

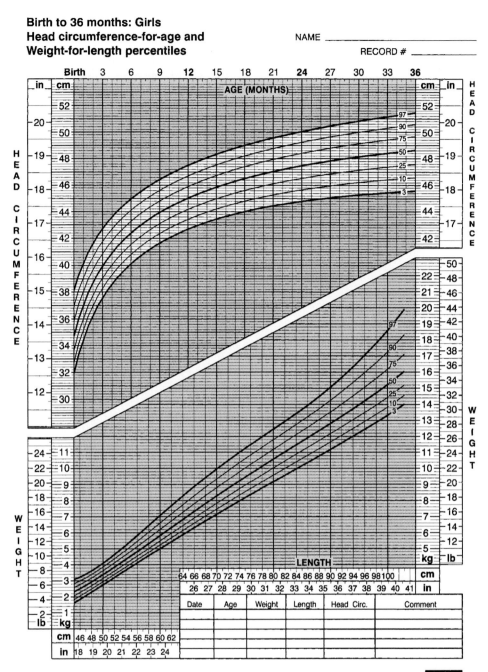

Birth to 36 months: Girls
Head circumference-for-age and
Weight-for-length percentiles

NAME _____

RECORD # _____

SOURCE: Developed by the National Center for Health Statistics in collaboration with
the National Center for Chronic Disease Prevention and Health Promotion (2000).
http://www.cdc.gov/growthcharts

CDC

FIGURE A-4 ◆

Physical growth percentiles for head circumference, weight for length—girls: birth to 36 months. From CDC, 2001.
www.cdc.gov/growthcharts

FIGURE A-5 ◆

Physical growth percentiles for stature and weight according to age—boys: 2 to 20 years. From CDC, 2001.

www.cdc.gov/growthcharts

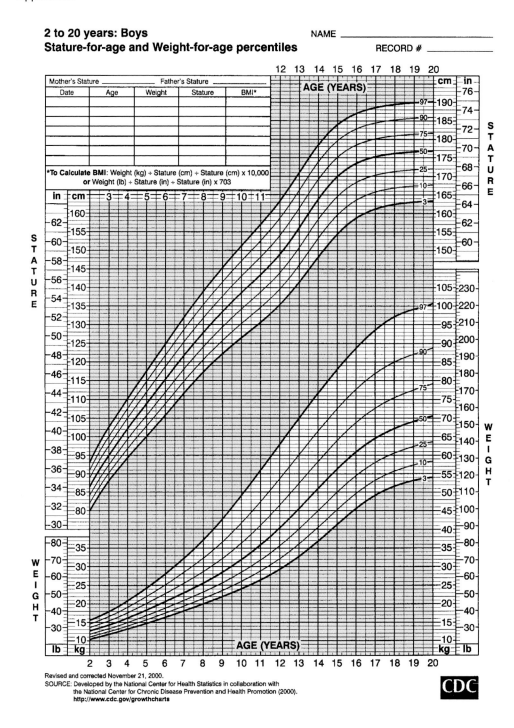

2 to 20 years: Boys
Stature-for-age and Weight-for-age percentiles

NAME _____

RECORD # _____

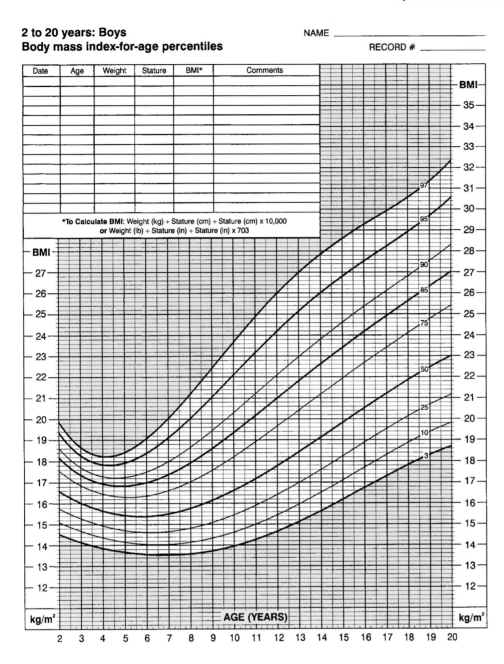

2 to 20 years: Boys
Body mass index-for-age percentiles

NAME _____

RECORD # _____

*To Calculate BMI: Weight (kg) ÷ Stature (cm) ÷ Stature (cm) x 10,000
or Weight (lb) ÷ Stature (in) ÷ Stature (in) x 703

SOURCE: Developed by the National Center for Health Statistics in collaboration with
the National Center for Chronic Disease Prevention and Health Promotion (2000).
http://www.cdc.gov/growthcharts

FIGURE A-6 ◆

Physical growth percentiles for body mass index according to age—boys: 2 to 20 years.
From CDC, 2001.
www.cdc.gov/growthcharts

FIGURE A-7 ◆

Physical growth percentiles for weight for stature—boys: 2 to 20 years.
From CDC, 2001.
www.cdc.gov/growthcharts

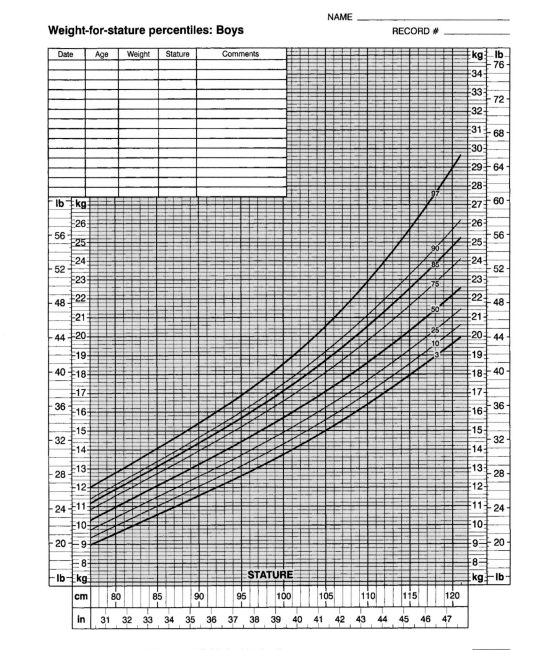

Weight-for-stature percentiles: Boys

SOURCE: Developed by the National Center for Health Statistics in collaboration with
the National Center for Chronic Disease Prevention and Health Promotion (2000).
http://www.cdc.gov/growthcharts

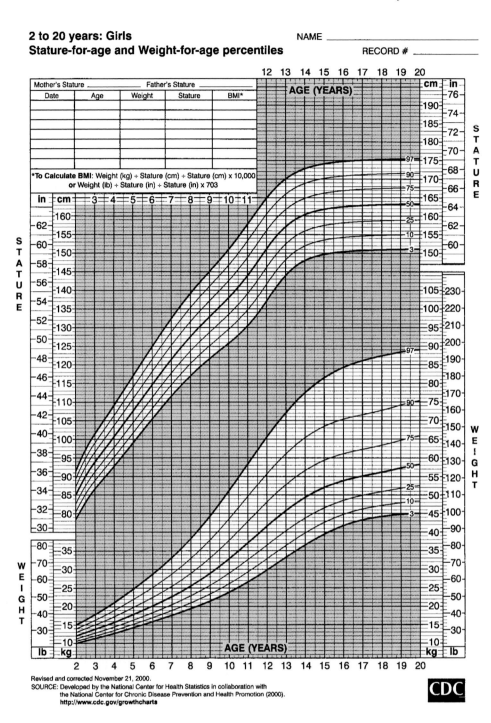

2 to 20 years: Girls
Stature-for-age and Weight-for-age percentiles

NAME _____

RECORD # _____

Revised and corrected November 21, 2000.
SOURCE: Developed by the National Center for Health Statistics in collaboration with
the National Center for Chronic Disease Prevention and Health Promotion (2000).
http://www.cdc.gov/growthcharts

FIGURE A-8 ◆

Physical growth percentiles for stature and weight according to age—girls: 2 to 20 years.
From CDC, 2001.
www.cdc.gov/growthcharts

FIGURE A-9 ◆

Physical growth percentiles for body mass index according to age—girls: 2 to 20 years. From CDC, 2001. *www.cdc.gov/growthcharts*

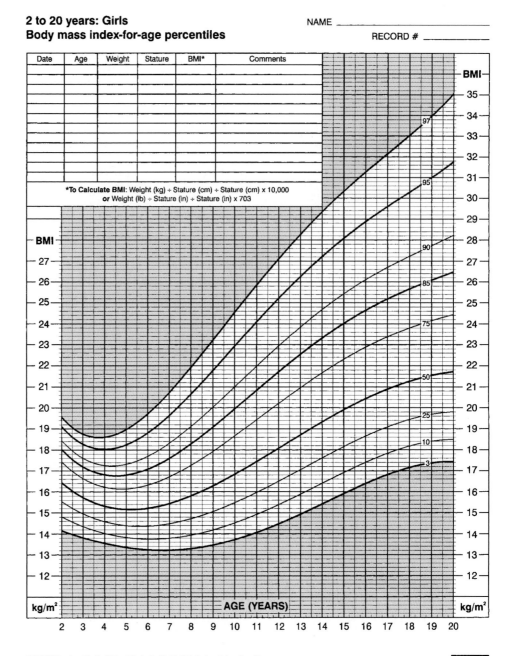

2 to 20 years: Girls
Body mass index-for-age percentiles

NAME _____

RECORD # _____

*To Calculate BMI: Weight (kg) ÷ Stature (cm) ÷ Stature (cm) x 10,000
or Weight (lb) ÷ Stature (in) ÷ Stature (in) x 703

SOURCE: Developed by the National Center for Health Statistics in collaboration with
the National Center for Chronic Disease Prevention and Health Promotion (2000).
http://www.cdc.gov/growthcharts

FIGURE A-10 ◆

Physical growth percentiles for weight for stature—girls: 2 to 20 years.
From CDC, 2001.
www.cdc.gov/growthcharts

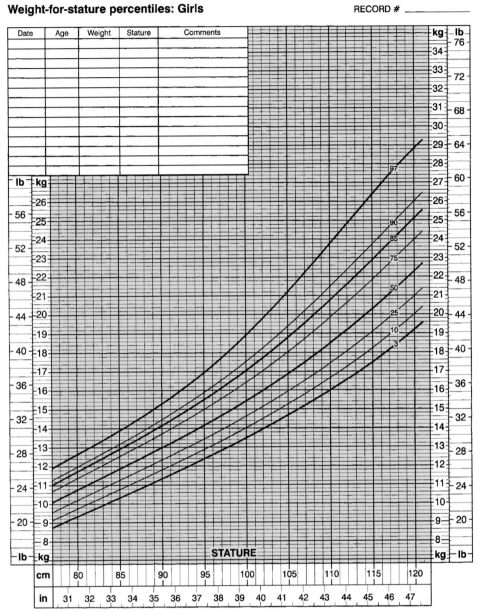

Weight-for-stature percentiles: Girls

NAME _____

RECORD # _____

STATURE

SOURCE: Developed by the National Center for Health Statistics in collaboration with the National Center for Chronic Disease Prevention and Health Promotion (2000).
http://www.cdc.gov/growthcharts

Appendix B: West Nomogram—Body Surface Area

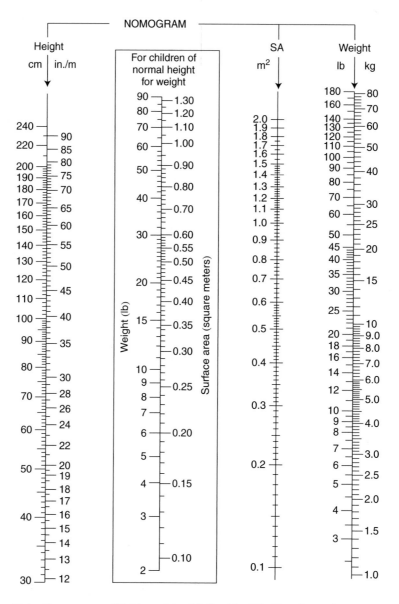

Note: *Nomogram modified from data of E. Boyd by C.D. West; from Behrman, R.E., Kliegman, R.M., & Jenson, H.B. (eds.). (2000).* Nelson textbook of pediatrics *(16th ed.). Philadelphia: W.B. Saunders.*

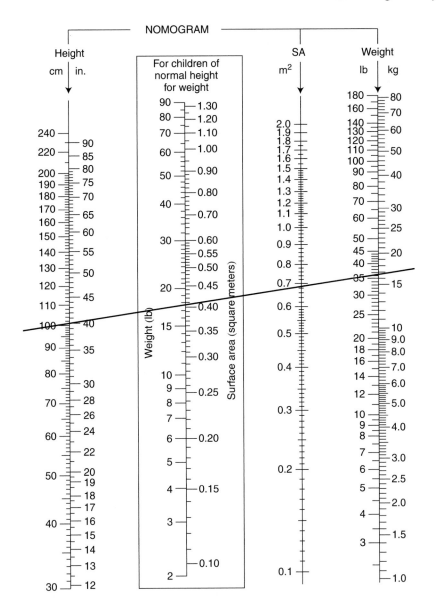

Pediatric doses of medications are generally based on body surface area (BSA) or weight. To calculate a child's BSA, draw a straight line from the height (in the left-hand column) to the weight (in the right-hand column). The point at which the line intersects the surface area (SA) column is the BSA (measured in square meters [m^2]). If the child is of roughly normal proportion, BSA can be calculated from the weight alone (in the enclosed area).

References

American Heart Association. (2000). 2000 guidelines for cardiopulmonary resuscitation and emergency cardiac care. *Circulation, 102*(Special Supplement), 1-384.

Berry, B.E., Simons, B.D., Siatkowski, R.M., Schiffman, J.C., Flynn, J.T. & Duthie, M.J. (2001). Preschool vision screening using the MTI-Photoscreener. *Pediatric Nursing 27*, 27-34.

Bukowski, T.P. & Freedman, A.L. (1999). Urethral catheterization: the case for caution. *Contemporary Pediatrics 16*, 100-115.

Dieckman, R., Brownstein, D., & Gaushe-Hill, M (eds.). (2000). *Pediatric Education for Prehospital Professionals*/American Academy of Pediatrics, Sudbury, MA: Jones and Barlett Publishers.

Eichelberger, M., Ball, J., Pratsch, G. & Clark, J. (1998). *Pediatric emergencies: a manual for pre-hospital care providers* (2nd ed.). Upper Saddle River, NJ: Prentice Hall.

Ellett, M.L. & Beckstrand, J. (1999). Examination of gavage tube placement in children. *Journal of the Society of Pediatric Nurses 4*, 51-60.

Ellett, M.L. & Beckstrand, J. (2001). Predicting the distance for Nasojejunal tube insertion in children. *Journal of the Society of Pediatric Nurses 6*, 123-132.

Fremgen, B.F. & Blume, W. (2001). *Phlebotomy basics: with other laboratory techniques*. Upper Saddle River, NJ: Prentice Hall.

Frey, A.M. & Schears, G. (2001). Dislodgment rates and impact of securement methods for peripherally inserted central catheters (PICCs) in children. *Pediatric Nursing 27*, 185-189.

Goodfellow, L.T., & Jones, M. (2002). Bronchial hygiene therapy. *American Journal of Nursing, 102*(1), 37-43.

Heilskov, J., Kleiber, C., Johnson, K. & Miller, J. (1998). A randomized trial of heparin and saline for maintaining intravenous locks in neonates. *Journal of the Society of Pediatric Nurses 3*, 111-116.

Joint Commisssion on Accreditation of Healthcare Organizations. (2001). *2001-2002 CAMHCN: Comprehensive Accreditation Manual for Health Care Networks Supplement*, Appendix D, http://www.jcaho.com/search_frm.html

Klein, T. (2001). PICCs and midlines—fine-tuning your care. *RN 64*, 26-29.

Metheny, N.A. & Titler, M.G. (2001). Assessing placement of feeding tubes. *American Journal of Nursing 101*(5), 36-46.

Mudge, B., Forcier, D. & Slattery, M.J. (1998). Patency of 24-gauge peripheral intermittent infusion devices: a comparison of heparin and saline flush solutions. *Pediatric Nursing 24*, 142-149.

O'Brien, B.K. (1999). Coming of age with an ostomy. *American Journal of Nursing 99*, 71-75.

Paisley, M.K., Stamper, M., Brown, J., Brown, N. & Ganong, L.H. (1997). The use of heparin and normal saline flushes in neonatal intravenous catheters. *Pediatric Nursing 23*, 521-527.

Passanza, C. (2001). Monitor options. *RN 64*(6), 34-41.

Prior, M. & Miles, S. (1999). Continuing professional development: casting: part one. *Emergency Nurse 7*, 33-42.

Racadio, J.M., Doellman, D.A., Johnson, N.D., Bean, J.A. & Jacobs, B.R. (2001). Pediatric peripherally inserted central catheters: complication rates related to catheter tip locations. *Pediatrics 107*, e28.

Richman, E. (1997). Asthma diagnosis and management: New severity classifications and therapy alternatives. *Clinician Reviews, 7*(8), 76–112.

Selekman, J. & Snyder, B. (1997). Institutional policies on the use of physical restraints on children. *Pediatric Nursing 23*, 531-537.

Smith, S.F. & Duell, D.J. (1996). *Clinical nursing skills, 4th Ed.* Stamford, CT: Appleton & Lange.

Swearingen, P.L. & Howard, C.A. (1996). *Photo atlas of nursing procedures*, 3rd Ed., Menlo Park, CA: Addison-Wesley.

Togger, D.A. & Brenner, P.S. (2001). Metered dose inhalers. *American Journal of Nursing 101*, 26-32.

Valencia, I.C., Falabella, A.F. & Schachner, LA. (2001). New developments in wound care for infants and children. *Pediatric Annals 30*, 211-218.

Winn, R. N. (2000). Oral meperidine, atropine, and pentobarbital for pediatric conscious sedation. *Pediatric Nursing 26*, 500-509.

Index